医画西游

主编／王珊珊

U0194182

全国百佳图书出版单位
中国中医药出版社
·北 京·

图书在版编目（CIP）数据

医画西游 / 王珊珊主编 .—北京：中国中医药出版社，2022.12
（医画四大名著）
ISBN 978-7-5132-8042-6

Ⅰ.①医…　Ⅱ.①王…　Ⅲ.①中国医药学—文化—
儿童读物　Ⅳ.① R2-05

中国国家版本馆 CIP 数据核字（2023）第 033963 号

中国中医药出版社出版
北京经济技术开发区科创十三街 31 号院二区 8 号楼
邮政编码　100176
传真　010-64405721
保定市中画美凯印刷有限公司印刷
各地新华书店经销

开本 889×1194　1/24　印张 3.75　字数 77 千字
2022 年 12 月第 1 版　2022 年 12 月第 1 次印刷
书号　ISBN 978-7-5132-8042-6

定价　29.90 元
网址　www.cptcm.com

服 务 热 线　010-64405510
购 书 热 线　010-89535836
维 权 打 假　010-64405753

微信服务号　zgzyycbs
微商城网址　https：//kdt.im/LIdUGr
官 方 微 博　http：//e.weibo.com/cptcm
天猫旗舰店网址　https：//zgzyycbs.tmall.com

编委会

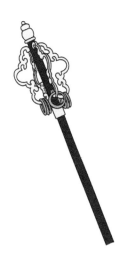

主　　编：王珊珊

副 主 编：孙熙蕊　杨雨滢　王乐鹏

编　　委：崔　悦　丁东宁　卢　佳　马亚茹

插画创作：谭茗月　陈家齐　陈乙漫　王　骁

　　　　　李姝靓　林舒婷

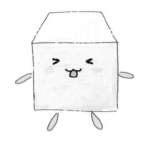

主编简介

　　王珊珊，英语语言文学硕士，中医诊断学在读博士，北京中医药大学人文学院副教授，硕士研究生导师；兼任世界中医药学会联合会翻译专业委员会理事，中国中医药研究促进会中医药翻译与国际传播专业委员会常务理事、传统文化翻译与国际传播专业委员会理事；研究方向为中医典籍翻译、中医国际传播。

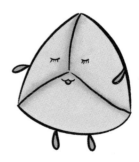

前　言

　　经典是古人智慧的结晶，蕴含着基本的价值观念与人生哲学。中国优秀传统思想文化体现着中华民族世世代代在生活中形成和传承的世界观、人生观、价值观等。中医药文化根植于中华传统文化，具有独特的魅力和文化意义。

　　中医药复兴与民族复兴密不可分，我们要传承中医药事业，发挥中医药在建设健康中国的作用。少年强则国强，中医药文化的传承自当从孩子抓起。

　　6~12 岁的孩子正处于观念与理念的塑形时期，接受新鲜事物较快，是文化、素质启蒙教育的最佳时期。在这一阶段学习传统中医药知识，有利于他们提高认知能力，培养中医传统思维方式，学会用理性的思维对待生活，用辩证的观念去处理生活和学习中遇到的问题。孩子若能了解、掌握并传承中医药优秀传统文化，中医药就有了立于不败之地的必备条件，中华民族就有了中医药的文化基因和基础。

四大名著作为中国文学史中的经典作品，影响了一代又一代的中国人。基于四大名著中的中医药知识，我们创作了"医画四大名著"系列绘本，取经典之精华，希望与孩子们一起在耳熟能详的故事中探寻中医药文化的宝库。该系列绘本共四册，《医画西游》为之开篇。

《西游记》是由明代小说家吴承恩创作的中国古代第一部浪漫主义长篇小说，主要描写了孙悟空、猪八戒、沙僧三人保护唐僧西行取经的故事，深受孩子们的喜爱。书中蕴含丰富的中医药文化元素，字里行间涉及医理、医德、中医典籍、诊脉、辨证施治、药材、药性分析、炮制、药效及中医专用器具等。如第一回《灵根育孕源流出 心性修持大道生》中有云：

"春采百花为饮食，夏寻诸果作生涯。秋收芋栗延时节，冬觅黄精度岁华。"诗中提到的黄精，是一种药食同源的中药材。第四十一回《心猿遭火败 木母被魔擒》中有云："五辆车儿合五行，五行生化火煎成。肝火能生心火旺，心火致令脾土平。脾土生金金化水，水能生木彻通灵。生生化化皆因火，火遍长空万物荣。"以此表明五行与人体脏腑之间的关系。孩子们可以通过阅读《西游记》了解中医药知识，这种方式既形象又有趣。

本册绘本中精选的六篇故事，均改编自《西游记》中的中医药相关情节。生动形象的原创插画与中医药文化相得益彰，全方位引起小读者的共鸣，让孩子们在轻松有趣的氛围中接触中医药文化。同时，每个故事配有中医药知识的拓展，或是介绍故事中提到的中药，或是介绍有关中医的基础理论知识，带领孩子们走进中医药文化的大门，在经典中感受中医药文化之美。

通过"医画四大名著"系列绘本，希望更多的小读者能够了解中医药，喜爱中医药，传承中医药，传播中医药。

王珊珊

2022 年 10 月

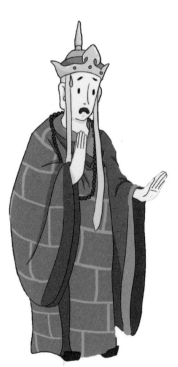

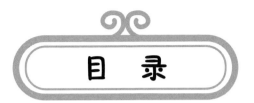

目 录

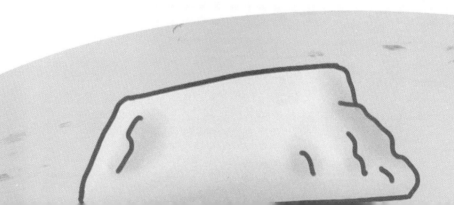

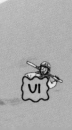

花果山采药记

传说在很久很久以前，在东胜神洲傲来国，有一座花果山，山上有一块仙石。一天，仙石崩裂，从中蹦出一只石猴来。石猴和一般猴子没什么区别，食草木，饮山泉，采山花，觅野果。

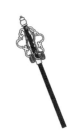

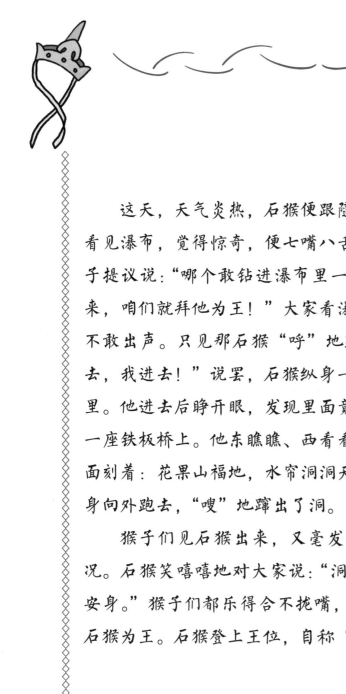

这天，天气炎热，石猴便跟随猴群到山涧里洗澡。猴子们看见瀑布，觉得惊奇，便七嘴八舌地议论起来。有只年长的猴子提议说："哪个敢钻进瀑布里一探究竟，又能安然无恙地出来，咱们就拜他为王！"大家看瀑布飞流直下，面面相觑，都不敢出声。只见那石猴"呼"地跳了出来，高声喊道："我进去，我进去！"说罢，石猴纵身一跃，一个跟头便翻进了瀑布里。他进去后睁开眼，发现里面竟一滴水也没有，自己正站在一座铁板桥上。他东瞧瞧、西看看，只见洞中有一块石碑，上面刻着：花果山福地，水帘洞洞天。石猴高兴得不得了，忙转身向外跑去，"嗖"地蹿出了洞。

猴子们见石猴出来，又毫发无损，都争着问他里面的情况。石猴笑嘻嘻地对大家说："洞里面没有水，正适合大伙儿安身。"猴子们都乐得合不拢嘴，随他进洞，又遵照诺言，拜石猴为王。石猴登上王位，自称"美猴王"。

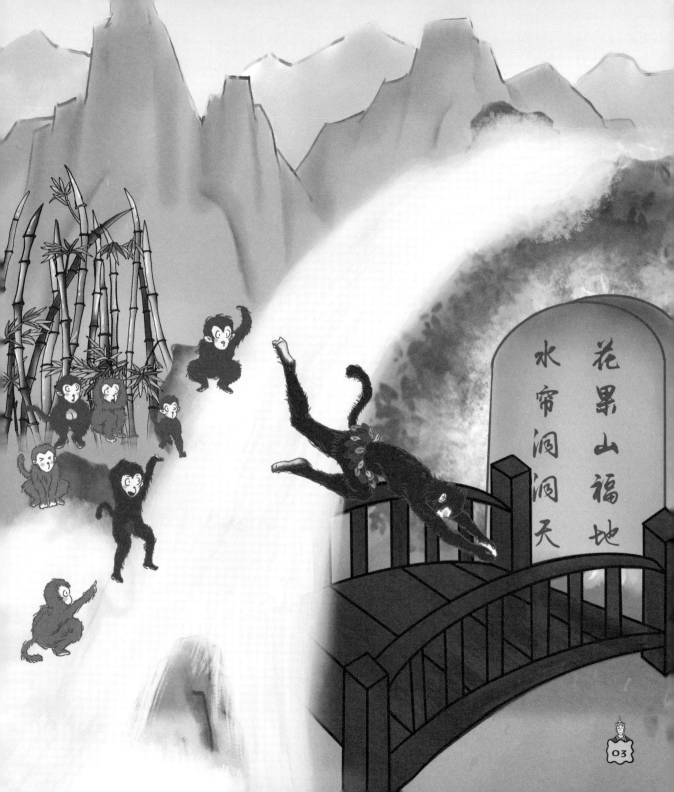

花果山福地
水帘洞洞天

03

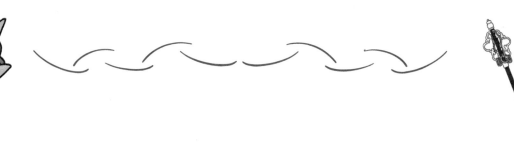

美猴王领一群猿猴、猕猴、马猴等，朝游花果山，暮宿水帘洞，是以——

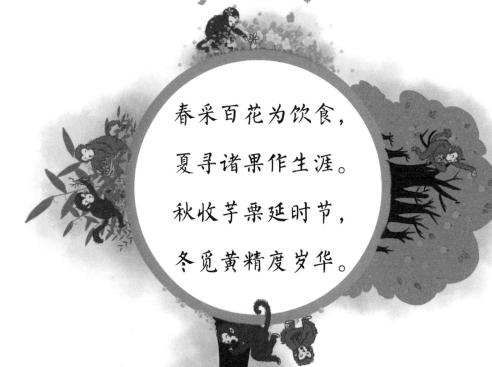

春采百花为饮食，
夏寻诸果作生涯。
秋收芋栗延时节，
冬觅黄精度岁华。

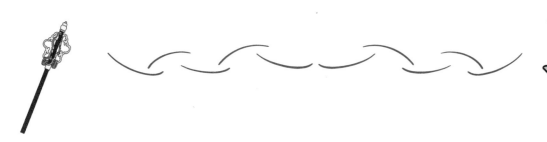

次日，众猴在美猴王的带领下去采仙桃、刨山药，回来之后煮烂黄精，捣碎薏苡仁和茯苓。猴子们吃得津津有味，问美猴王："这是什么好东西呀？"美猴王拿起黄精说："你们看，这是黄精，可以补中益气、养阴润肺、健脾补肾。猴伯伯腰膝酸软，没有力气，吃这个就会恢复体力了。"

黄 精

黄精是一种药食同源的中药材，具有补气养阴、健脾、润肺、益肾之功效。中医学理论认为"腰为肾之府"，伴随着年龄的增大，许多老年人会出现肾虚的现象，肾气亏虚则腰府中空，肌肉得不到濡润，所以家里的爷爷奶奶经常会发生腰酸腿痛的情况。

文中的猴伯伯正是通过吃黄精补肾，缓解了腰膝酸软的症状。同时，黄精泡水喝还能起到补血作用。然而黄精也不宜吃太多，因为黄精性质滋腻，食用过多会增加脾胃负担。

这时，远处忽然传来一阵哭闹声，美猴王过去一看，原来是一只小猴子闹着不吃饭。小猴揞着肿得高高的小腿，说自己吃不下饭、睡不好觉。

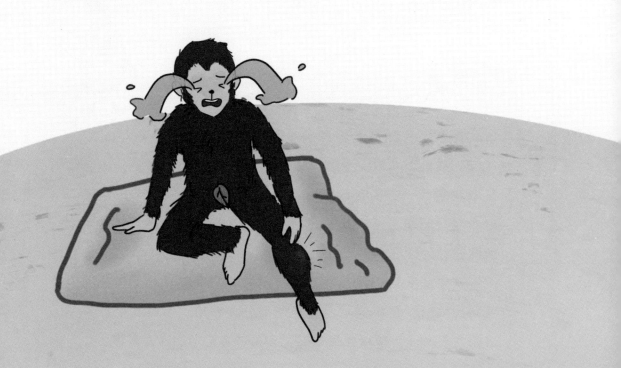

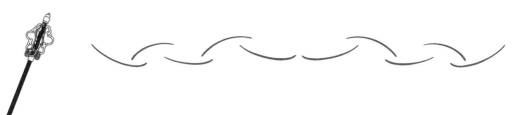

　　美猴王忙给他喂了茯苓和薏苡仁，说："这是患了水肿。别害怕，吃了这两味利水渗湿、健脾宁心的药，很快就会好的。"果然，小猴子小腿上的肿很快消了下去，从此以后吃得香、睡得香，又能开开心心地和大家一起玩耍了。

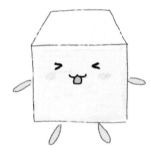

茯　苓

　　茯苓又称玉灵、松薯等，具有健脾、宁心、利尿的功效。小猴子吃了茯苓，通过增加尿量来排出体内多余的水分，水肿就消除了！小朋友要注意，茯苓利尿的作用十分显著，服用茯苓过量会导致排尿次数增多。

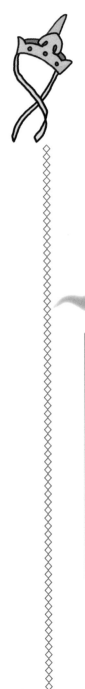
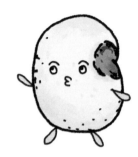

薏苡仁

薏苡仁，也就是薏米，是我国传统的药食同源保健食品。薏苡仁和茯苓一样，不仅能利尿消肿，还有健脾祛湿、增强免疫力等功效。

薏苡仁和茯苓的健脾功能很受推崇。脾为五脏之一，脾主运化，喜燥恶湿。住在潮湿之地的人们经常用薏苡仁和茯苓煲汤或者熬粥，通过加强脾胃的运化功能来除去体内的湿气。此外医书古籍均有记载，经常食用薏苡仁可以使皮肤细腻润滑、白皙有光泽。

齐天大圣大闹天宫

话说这孙悟空在花果山好吃好喝，养得身强体壮，又仗着一身本领，大闹龙宫和地府，无法无天。阎王和龙王都去找玉皇大帝告状。太白金星给玉皇大帝出了个主意，说不如随便给他一个官职，把他放在眼皮子底下，于是玉皇大帝让孙悟空去看马。然而"纸包不住火"，孙悟空发现这个官职竟然是最小的，一气之下奔回花果山，自封"齐天大圣"。

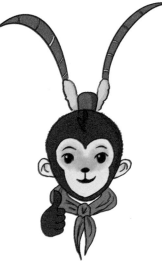

玉皇大帝听说孙悟空又回到花果山，马上命令托塔李天王和哪吒三太子带兵前去捉拿孙悟空。没想到天兵天将都败下阵来，太白金星只好又出了个主意："既然那猴子喜欢，不如就让他做个有名无权的齐天大圣！"玉皇大帝听了之后觉得有道理，即刻派太白金星去讲和。

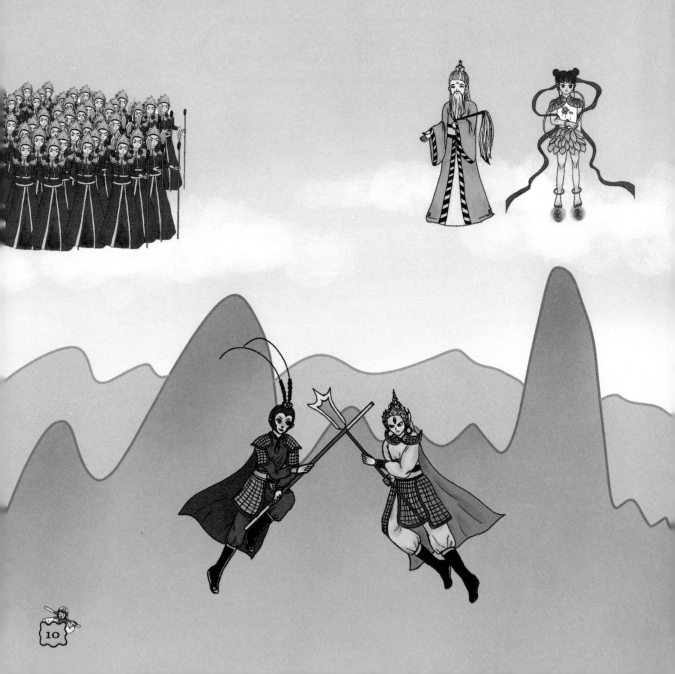

太白金星奉命来到花果山，宣读圣旨，大圣听后欣然同意，跟太白金星返回天宫。时间久了，玉皇大帝怕大圣闲着没事添麻烦，就让他去管蟠桃园。

谁知大圣趁王母娘娘寿宴之际，竟大胆偷吃了园里的蟠桃，还大闹蟠桃会，闯下了大祸，随后又跑回花果山去了。玉皇大帝知道后，勃然大怒，命人下凡，将这泼猴儿捉拿回了天庭。

大圣虽被绑在斩妖台上，但却刀枪不入、水火不侵，众神仙不论使什么法子，都不能伤他一根毫毛。束手无策之际，太上老君灵机一动，提议道："那妖猴既是天地灵物，又吃了不少蟠桃、仙丹等好东西，已成了金刚之躯，不如把他扔进我的炼丹炉中炼化成丹！"正为此事焦头烂额的玉皇大帝，闻言立刻准奏。

大圣就这样被押入了老君的炼丹炉里，炙热的炉火让大圣急得到处乱蹦。烧火的童子使出了九牛二虎之力，煽风助火，欲借六丁神火尽快炼化了那猴儿。

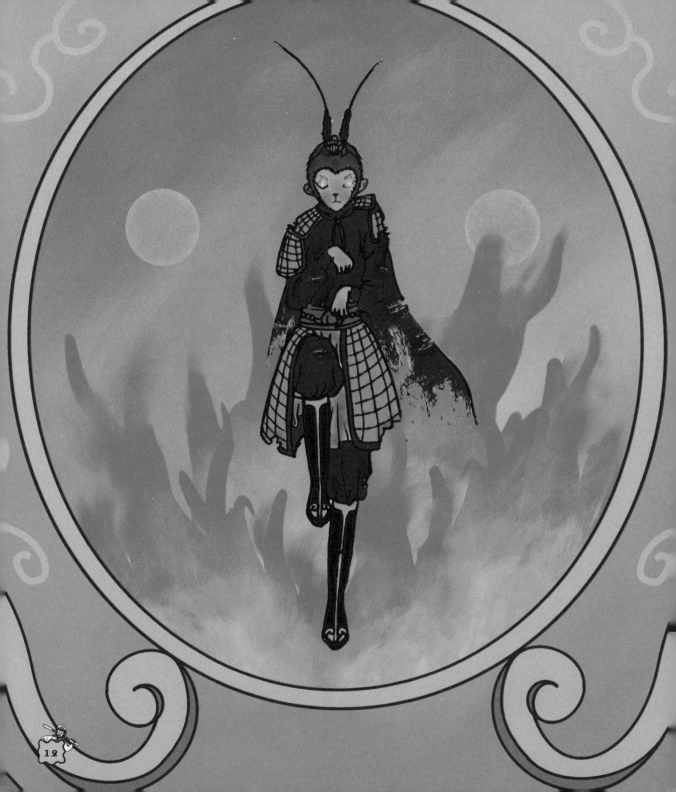

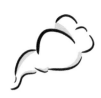

　　七七四十九天过去了，炉中早已没了动静，太上老君信心满满地打开炉门，却见有什么东西从炉里蹦了出来，竟是那早该被炼化的大圣！

　　原来那八卦炉是乾、坎、艮、震、巽、离、坤、兑八卦。正所谓："天无绝人之路！"大圣在炉中跳来跳去时，无意间跳到了巽宫的位置，八卦中巽为风，故此地只有烟没有火。大圣就这样蹲在巽宫躲了四十九天，竟把双眼熏成了"火眼金睛"。

　　大圣跳出炼丹炉，将其踢倒，抢起如意棒，直打到灵霄殿上。

　　玉皇大帝无奈，只好派人去西天请如来佛祖。大圣此时怒气冲冲。

　　如来佛祖不急不恼，微笑着摊开手掌说："你敢不敢和我打一个赌？如果你有本事一筋斗翻出我的手掌，我就让玉皇大帝把位子给你。"

　　大圣一个筋斗云就能翻出

十万八千里，志在必得，喊道："一言既出，驷马难追！我去了，你可别反悔！"说着，他翻了个筋斗便无影无踪了。

大圣腾云驾雾，不知过了多久，只见眼前出现了五根通天的柱子，这才停下，心想："这五根柱子一定是撑天用的，想必我这是到天边了吧！"

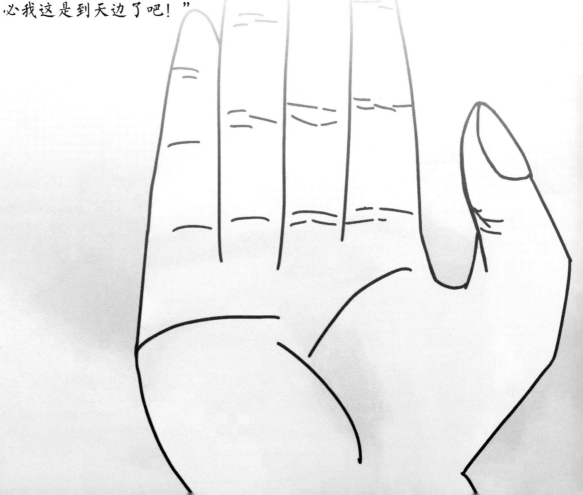

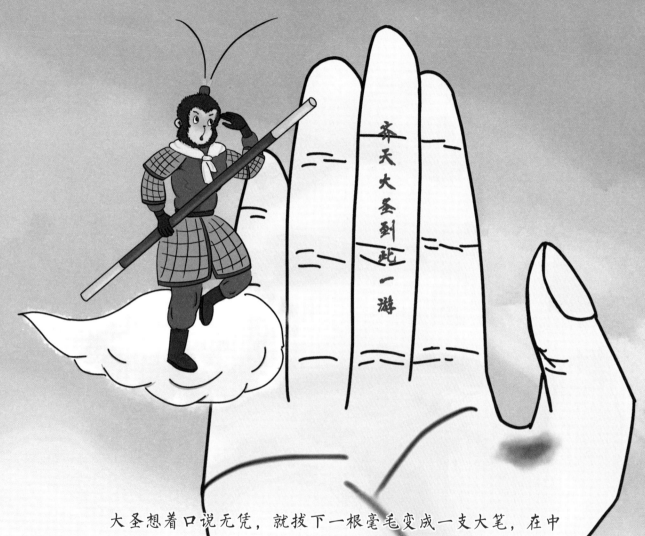

大圣想着口说无凭，就拔下一根毫毛变成一支大笔，在中间的一根柱子上写下"齐天大圣到此一游"八个大字。写完后，他又跑到第一根柱子下撒了一泡猴尿，这才又驾起筋斗云，飞回到如来佛祖面前。

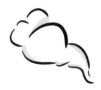

大圣得意地喊道："如来，说话算数！快叫玉皇大帝老儿让位子吧！"

如来佛祖却说大圣根本没有离开过他的掌心。大圣不服，要如来去看看他在天边留下的证据。如来佛祖让大圣看看他右手的中指，再闻闻大拇指根。大圣睁大金睛火眼，只见佛祖右手中指上有他写的那八个歪歪扭扭的大字，大拇指上还有些猴尿的臊气。

齐天大圣到此一游

大圣吃惊地说："我不信，一定是你使诈。我明明把字写在了撑天的柱子上，怎么会在你手上？等我去看看再说！"

大圣转身想跑，如来佛祖眼疾手快，反手一扑，把大圣推出西天门外，又把手的五指分别化作金、木、水、火、土五座联山，将大圣牢牢压在山下。这座联山便是"五行山"。

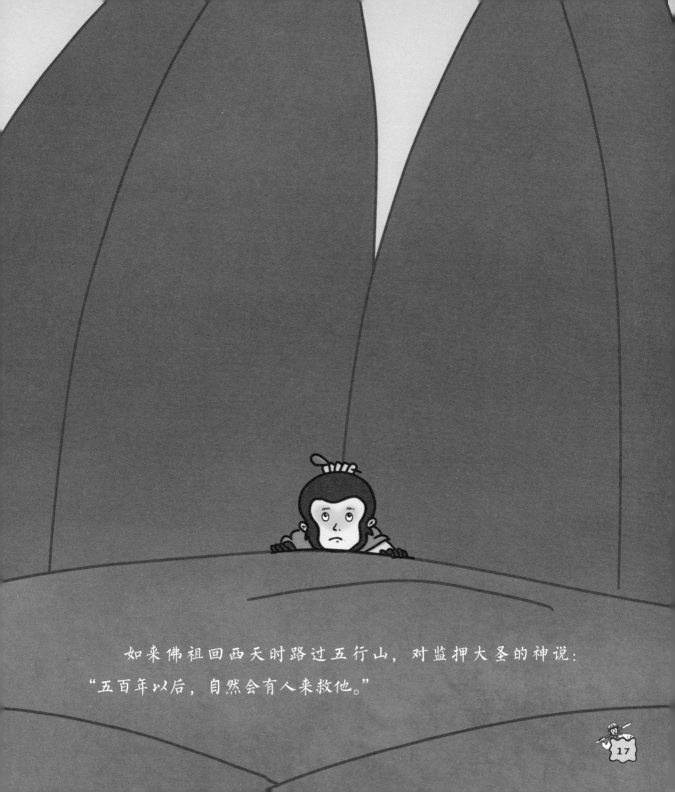

　　如来佛祖回西天时路过五行山，对监押大圣的神说："五百年以后，自然会有人来救他。"

五　行

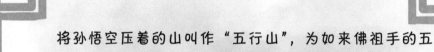

　　将孙悟空压着的山叫作"五行山"，为如来佛祖手的五指所化，分别为金、木、水、火、土这五座联山。

　　五行学说是中医基础理论之一，是中国古代哲学在认识自然界时所提出的概念。五行学说将宇宙万物划分为五种性质，即木、火、土、金、水，它们具有各自的功能和属性。木有生长、升发的特性，火有温热、向上的特性，土有承载、养育万物的特性，金有沉降、收敛的特性，水有滋润、寒凉的特性。

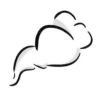
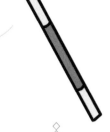

中医也将五行运用到人体上，以五行配五脏为例：

肝气升发属木，
心阳温煦属火，
脾主运化属土，
肺清肃下降属金，
肾藏精纳气属水。

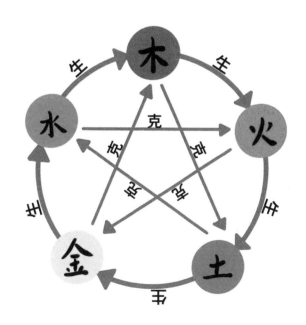

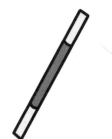

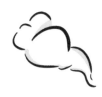

在五行理论中，根据五脏与五行的对应关系，推导出许多理论。金、木、水、火、土，在人体中分别对应肺、肝、肾、心、脾五脏。

金对应肺，肺与呼吸道疾病相关，如有呼吸急促、胸闷、咳嗽、语音低微等症状时，需要从肺治疗。

金

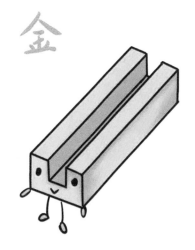

木

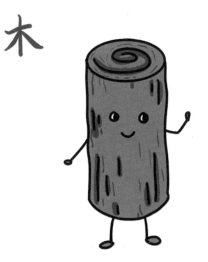

木对应肝，肝开窍于目，如有情绪易激动、烦躁不宁、胸胁隐痛、视力急剧下降等症状时，需要从肝治疗。

水对应肾，肾为先天之本，如有腰膝酸软、水肿、尿频、记忆力减退、无故大量脱发等症状时，需要从肾治疗。

　　火对应心，心主血脉，如有胸闷、失眠、健忘、烦躁，甚至心前区疼痛等症状时，需要从心治疗。

　　土对应脾，脾主肌肉，如有恶心呕吐、食欲不振、腹痛腹胀、四肢乏力等症状时，需要从脾治疗。

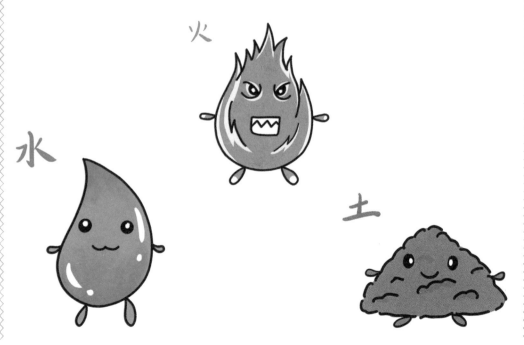

悟空风眼得妙药

话说唐僧从五行山下救出了孙悟空，又在高老庄收了二徒弟猪八戒，师徒三人不辞辛苦，日夜兼程地朝西天赶路。

正当他们翻山越岭之时，突然有一只猛虎跳了出来，喊道："来者何人？此处是黄风大王的地盘，我是虎先锋，奉大王之命来巡山！"师徒三人说明来历，请他放行。

谁知这妖精早就听闻吃了唐僧肉能长生不老的传言，一心想捉拿唐僧立功。他二话不说，就和八戒、悟空打了起来，却不是两人的对手，很快就落了下风。

虎先锋为了脱身，用爪子剥下

虎皮铺在石头上扮成自己，然后化作一股狂风溜走了。他逃跑时发现了落单的唐僧，大笑道："真是天助我也！"唐僧就这样被抓到洞中，献给了黄风大王。

悟空和八戒没能识破虎先锋的诡计，见那只老虎趴在石头上，一棍打下去，虎皮却化作了一股黑烟飘散，哪里还有虎先锋的影子。悟空一拍脑袋，懊悔地说："不好，咱们中了那妖精的调虎离山之计！"两人急忙回到原处，却怎么也寻不见师父的踪影。

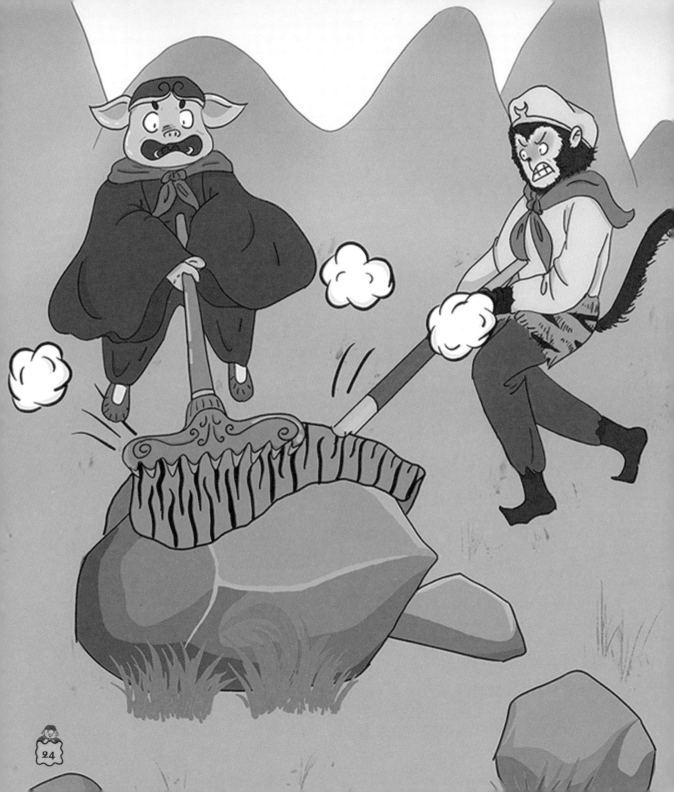

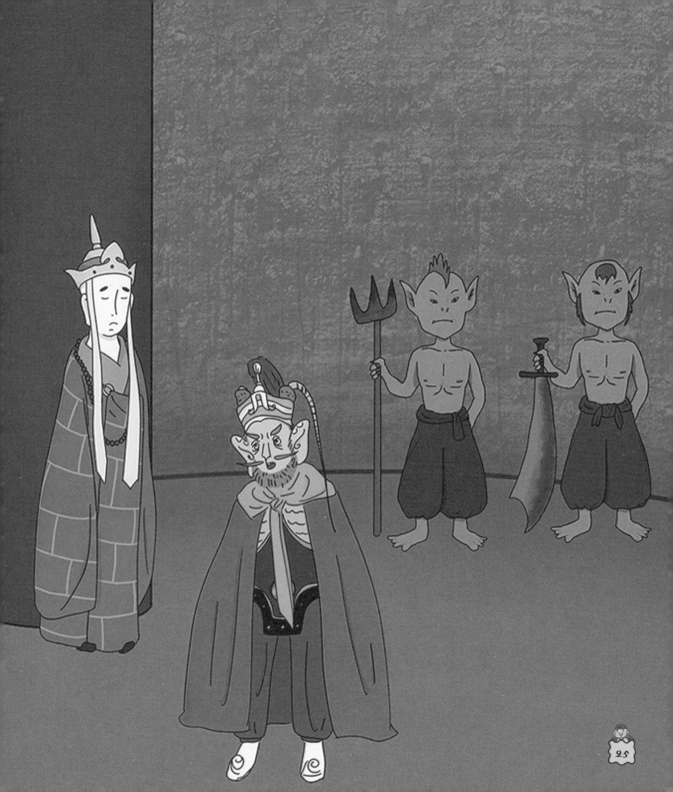

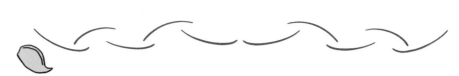

　　师兄弟两人追进山中，苦苦探寻，终于找到了妖洞门口。悟空让八戒看着马和行李，自己到洞口叫阵。黄风怪冲出洞口，与悟空斗了三十多个回合，仍不见胜负，便想暗算悟空。只见黄风怪猛地朝悟空脸上吹了口气，悟空顿时觉得双眼剧痛不已，仿佛被无数个针尖猛扎，疼得睁不开，立刻败下阵来。黄风怪趁机收兵，悟空也只好作罢。

　　败退的师兄弟二人借宿于山下的一位老人家里，老人热情

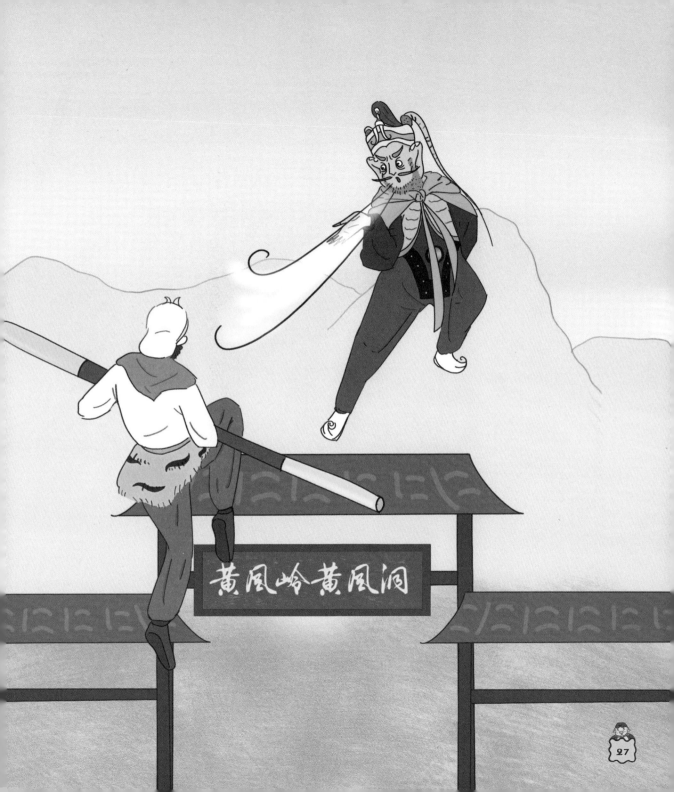

黄風嶺黄風洞

27

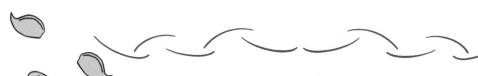

地招待了他们。老人见悟空不停地揉眼睛，十分痛苦的模样，便主动问起。八戒唉声叹气地说道："山上那妖怪朝我师兄的眼里吹了股妖风，我师兄便成了这副模样！老人家，您可有办法？"

老人家说："这是得了风眼啊！那妖怪口中喷出的是风热之气，也叫风火之邪。如果不彻底治好，以后恐怕会落下迎风流泪的毛病呢。"

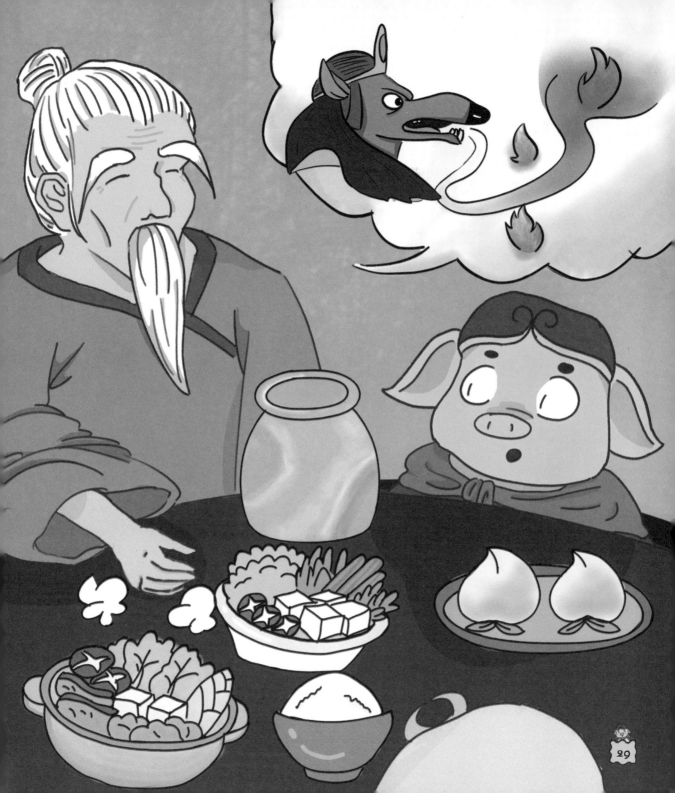

悟空急得抓耳挠腮，问道："俺老孙没了这火眼金睛可不行。现在可如何是好？"

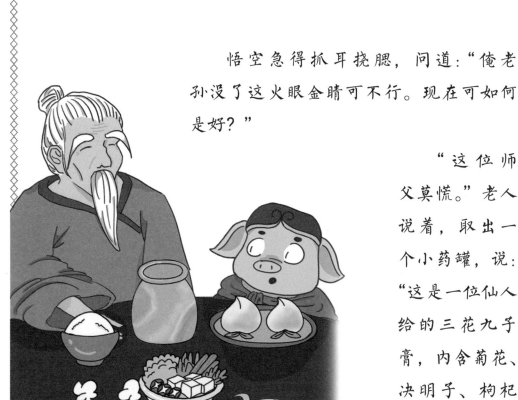

"这位师父莫慌。"老人说着，取出一个小药罐，说："这是一位仙人给的三花九子膏，内含菊花、决明子、枸杞子等解毒明目之药，专治一切风眼。"

悟空上了药，倒头便睡，第二天一睁眼，发现眼睛已经不痛不痒、恢复如初了。这时，悟空和八戒发现房子和老人都不见了。原来，这山中老人是菩萨派来暗中帮助他们的神仙！于是悟空前去南海求助菩萨，借来定风珠等宝物，降服黄风怪，把师父救了出来。

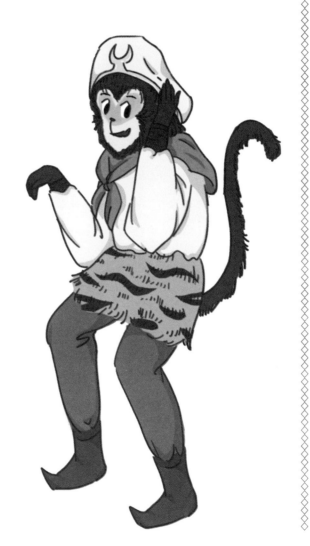

六淫

六淫中的"六"指的是风、寒、暑、湿、燥、火六种气候变化,"淫"指的是太多、太过。六种气候变化太过,便成为侵犯人体的外邪,损害人体健康。比如夏天的气温比较高,一般情况下,人体可以抵挡暑热,不会引发疾病。但如果长时间在太阳下暴晒,暑气就变成了暑邪,容易使人中暑,出现头晕、恶心甚至昏迷等症状。六淫的致病特点各不相同,因此熟悉六淫的症状有助于我们准确辨明病因。

悟空所受的风热之气中，风邪是导致生病的主要原因。风为"六邪之首"，很多疾病都是由风邪导致的，它还常常和其他邪气合并伤害人体，比如悟空所受的外邪是风邪夹杂热邪。如果小朋友在寒冷的天气吹冷风，就很容易得风寒感冒。所以小朋友们一定要好好锻炼身体，提高免疫力，避免遭受风邪之气。

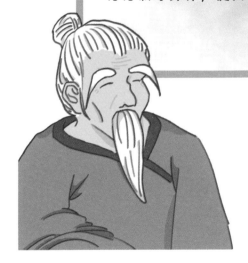

美味人参果

　　话说悟空治好眼睛后，很快打败了黄风怪，救出唐僧，继续赶路。一路上，唐僧又收了沙僧为三弟子。这天，师徒四人来到万寿山五庄观，想在这里借住一晚。五庄观里的两个道童一听他们自报家门，连忙恭敬地将四人迎了进去，说："我家师父讲经去了，让我们在这里等您，高僧快快请进！"唐僧细问才知道，原来这童子的师父是镇元子，与自己是五百年前的故交。

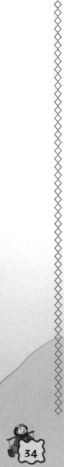

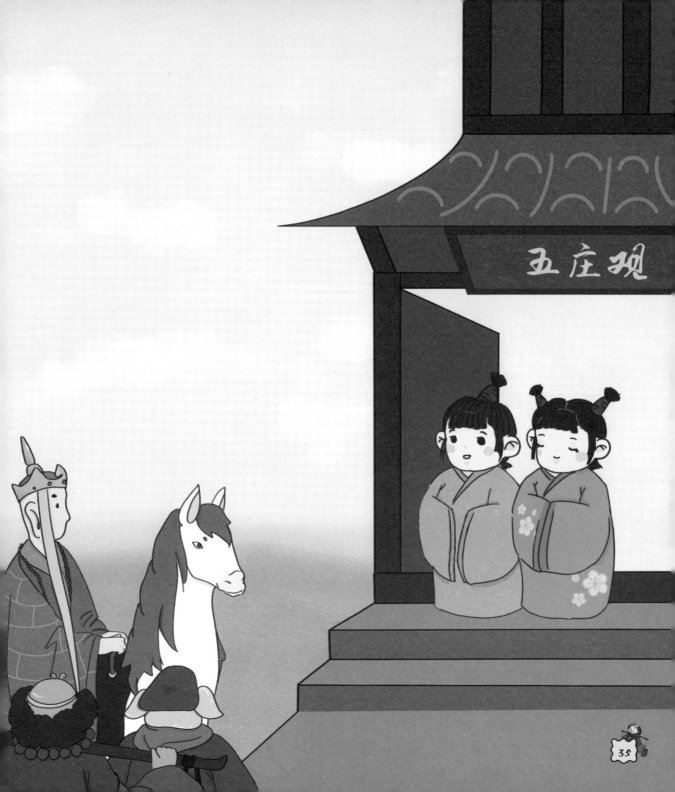

五庄观

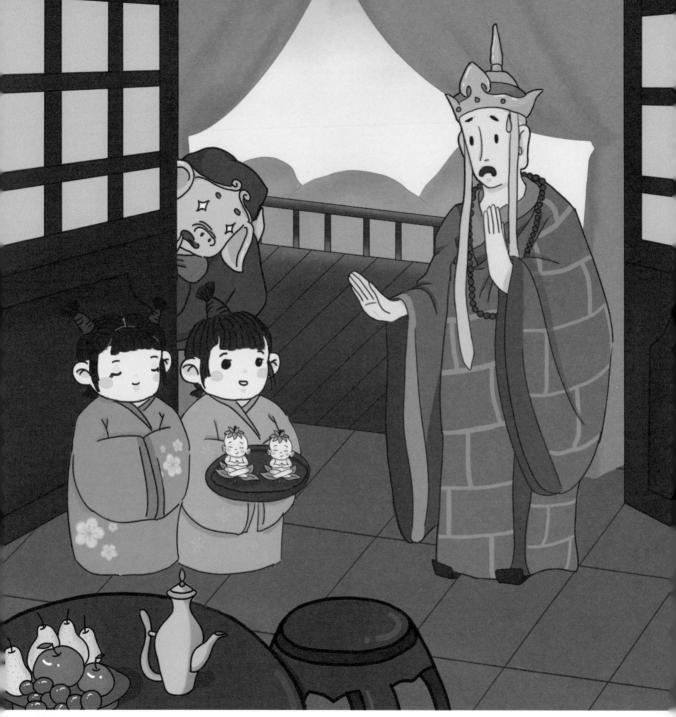

二童对唐僧礼遇有加，还特地摘了人参果给唐僧解渴。唐僧见人参果的形状像婴儿一般，连连摇头，不敢吃。两个童子解释说这是树上结的果子，可是唐僧偏不相信。两个童子见唐僧不吃，只好回到房里，分吃了人参果。

没想到，这件事却被嘴馋的八戒看到了。等悟空回来，八戒连忙把刚才的事情告诉了师兄，问："这人参果有什么好的呀？我听那两个童子说这是仙果。"悟空答道："这人参果可是延年益寿的好东西。"八戒听了垂涎三尺，连忙恳求师兄："这可是个难得的好东西呀！猴哥儿本事最大，你去摘几个，让师弟们也尝尝鲜！"

悟空偷拿了童子摘果用的金击子，跑到后园去摘人参果。他跳上树枝，用金击子一敲，那果子就掉落在地上没了踪影。

悟空断定是土地神贪嘴偷吃，不分青红皂白地把果园里的土地神抓来，逼他交出人参果。

土地神连呼冤枉，解释道："大圣有所不知，这果子中藏着五行的学问。它遇金而落，遇木而枯，遇水而化，遇火而焦，遇土而入。敲时要用金器，才能击落。若这果子落在地上，便自己钻入地里了。"悟空恍然大悟，一手拿金击子敲，一手扯着自己的衣服兜住三个果子。

38

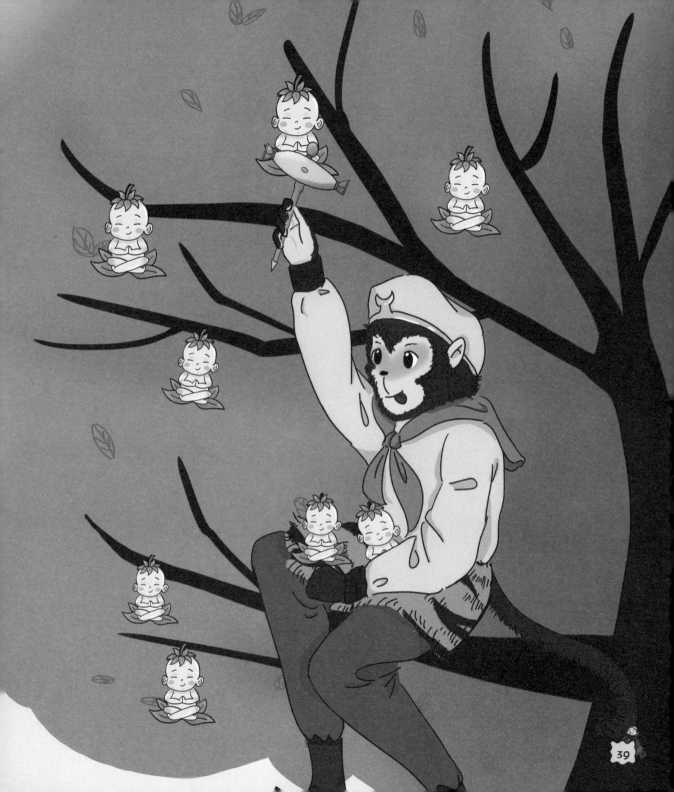

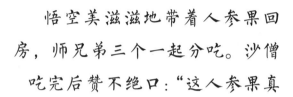

悟空美滋滋地带着人参果回房，师兄弟三个一起分吃。沙僧吃完后赞不绝口："这人参果真是香甜解渴啊。"不料没过多久，他们偷吃人参果的事就被发现了。两个道童对师徒四人破口大骂，悟空气不过，一怒之下推倒了人参果树。这时镇元子回来，看到宝树被毁，非常生气，可是念及自己与唐僧是故交，又知道悟空本领高强，也就不再为难他们，只要求悟空把树救活。

悟空问遍各路神仙，都没找到治活人参果树的办

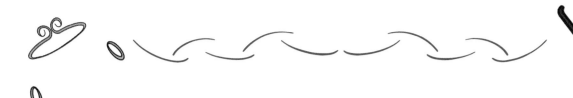

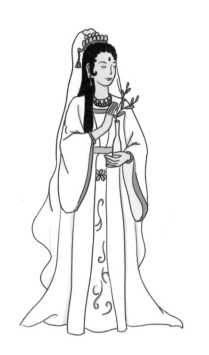

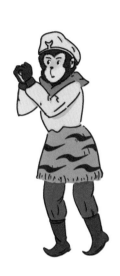

法。最后，他只好去找观音菩萨帮忙。幸运的是，观音手中玉净瓶里的甘露水正好能医治仙树仙草。

于是，悟空和观音菩萨一起驾云来到五庄观。观音菩萨让悟空师兄弟三人把树扛起来、扶正，用土把根埋上，然后一边念动咒语，一边用杨柳枝沾甘露水洒在树上。没过多久，那树的叶子也绿了，果子也长出来了，人参果树恢复了原样。

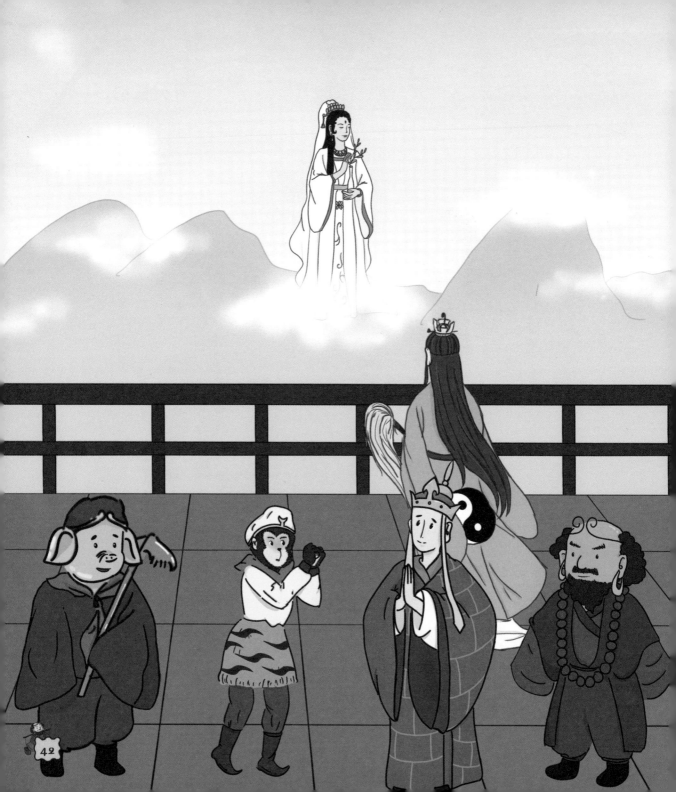

42

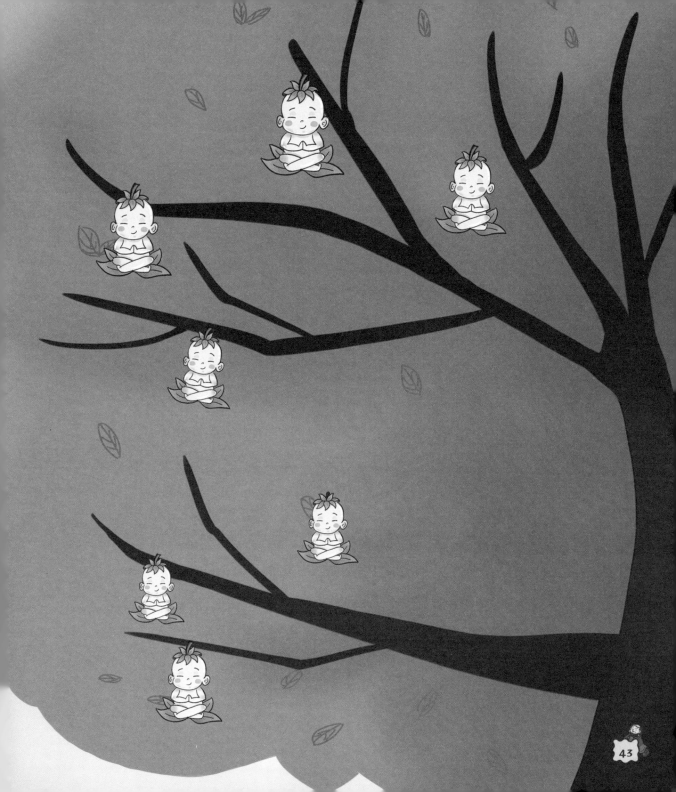

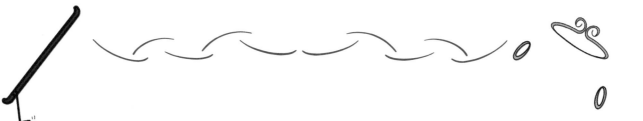

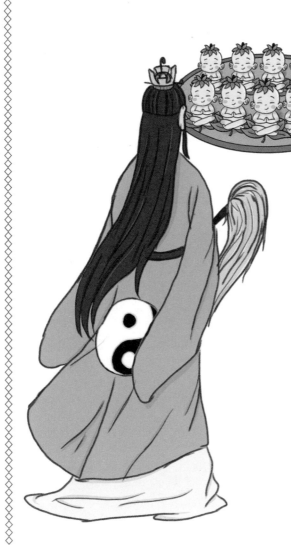

　　镇元子见树被救活，转怒为喜，立即让仙童敲下十个人参果来，请大家一起参加"人参果大会"。唐僧这时才明白这确实是果子，便吃了一个。散席后，镇元子送别唐僧师徒，四人继续西行。

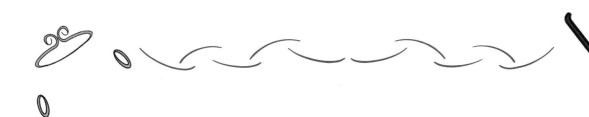

人参果

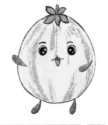

　　故事中的人参果和我们现在食用的人参果不一样。这里的人参果长得像孩童，能够补精气、壮元神、延年益寿、生津止渴。而现实中的人参果是球形的，原名为香瓜茄，又名长寿果，是一种营养较为全面的蔬果两用食品，其果实脆嫩、爽甜多汁、清香味美，含有丰富的维生素、蛋白质和钙，具有保健价值。

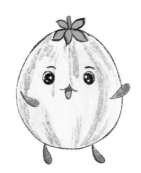

大战红孩儿

唐僧师徒又行了半个月，这一日来到一座怪石嶙峋的大山前。山前忽然飞沙走石，迷住了师徒四人的眼睛。待狂风停歇，唐僧已不见了踪影。师兄弟三人急忙四处探查，才知这山中有一处火云洞，洞中住着一只妖怪，名叫红孩儿。原来这红孩儿听说吃了唐僧肉能长生不老，想孝敬父母牛魔王和铁扇公主，便施法召来风沙，趁机把唐僧给抓走了。

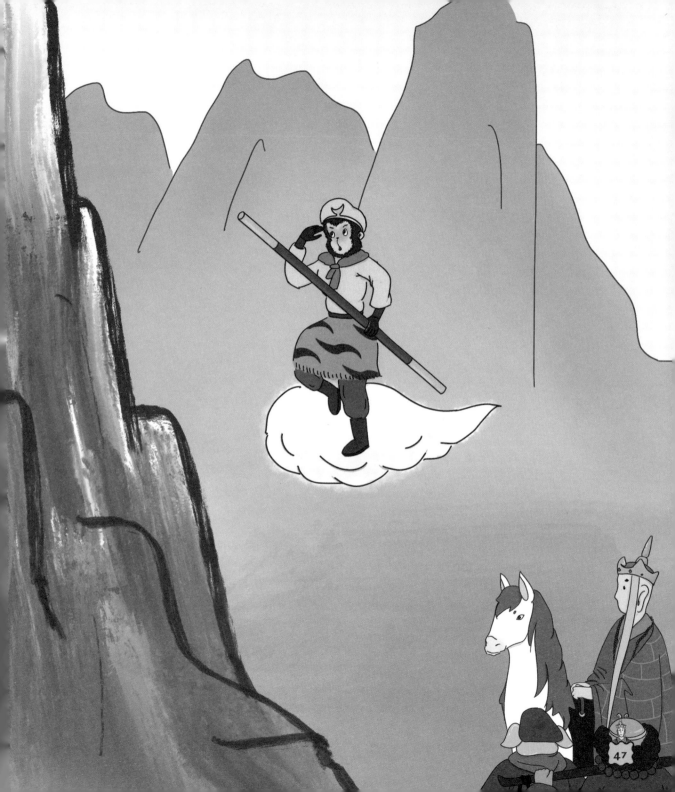

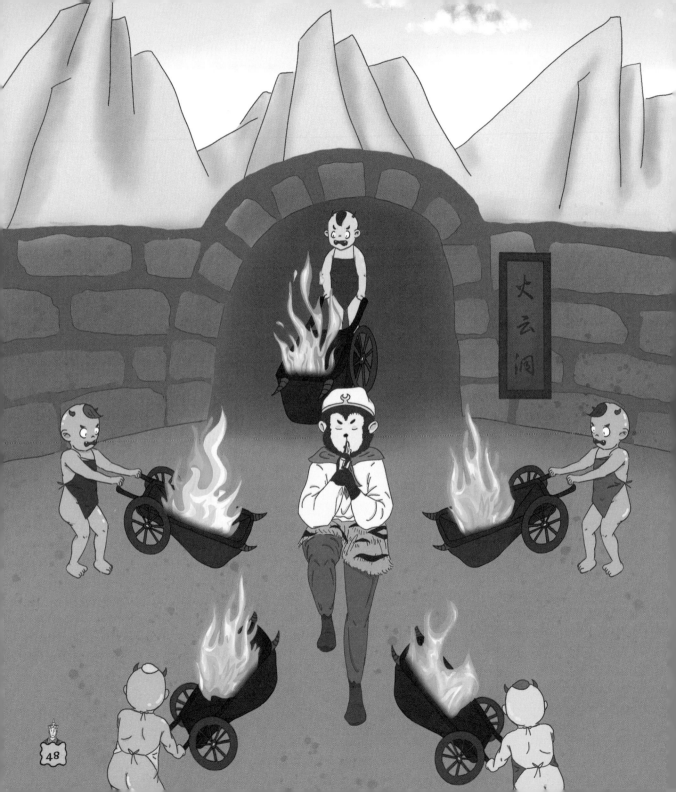

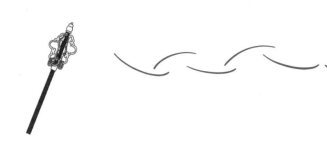
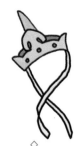

三人即刻动身，去火云洞前叫阵。只见洞中涌出一群小妖，小妖们推出五辆车子，按照金、木、水、火、土的顺序摆成法阵，车上顿时火光四起，火云洞烟雾弥漫。

悟空艺高人胆大，施了一道避火诀就往火里闯。不料，这火并非普通的野火，而是红孩儿修炼的三昧真火！烈火里浓烟滚滚，悟空什么也看不见，只得无功而返。

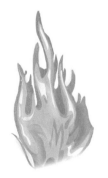
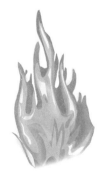
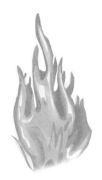

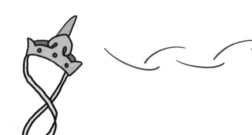
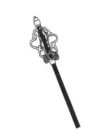
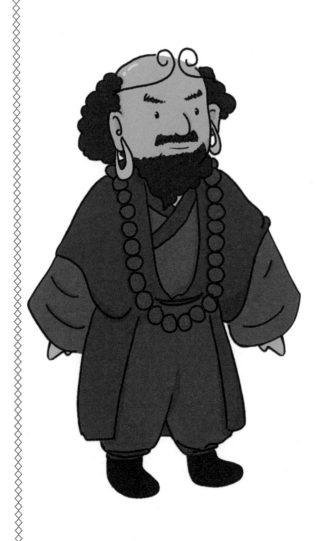

师兄弟三人一时束手无策。突然，沙僧提醒说："红孩儿擅长火攻，不如用五行相生相克的道理来治他。"悟空听后大喜："师弟说的有理！五行中水能克火，待俺去借水来，灭灭这妖怪的威风！"

悟空请来了四海龙王助阵。只见火云洞前大雨倾盆，可雨水落在三昧真火上，反而像火上浇油一样，越浇越旺了。

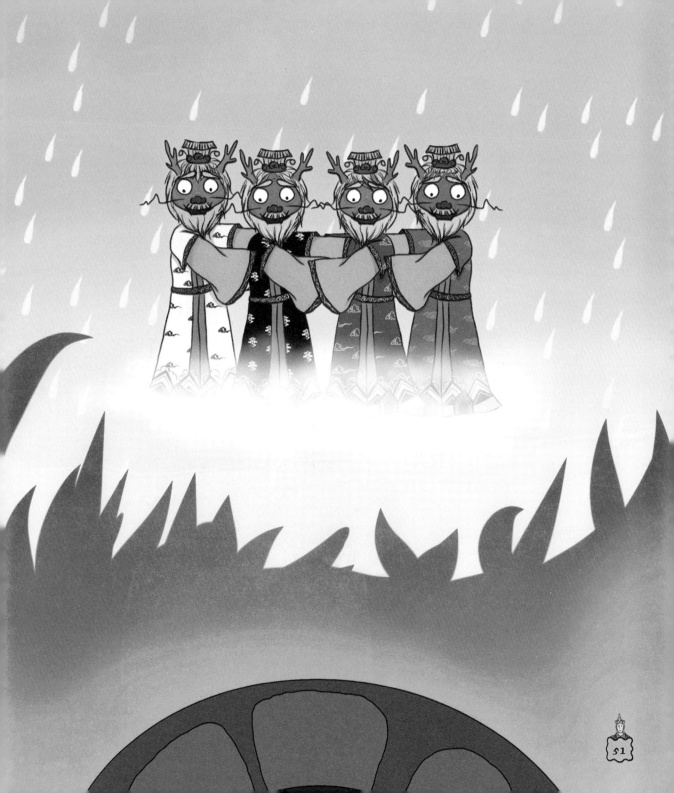

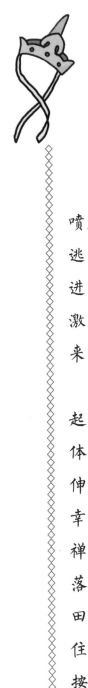
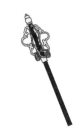

悟空担忧师父，忍不住冲进火里，却被那妖怪一口浓烟喷在脸上，熏得头晕眼花，分不清东南西北。他昏头昏脑地逃出洞去，一头栽进河里，被冷水一激，一口气没接上来，便不省人事了。

八戒、沙僧救起悟空，却见他身体蜷缩，四肢无法伸展，全身冰冷。幸好八戒懂得按摩禅法，知道悟空因落入冷水而气阻丹田。他将手搓热捂住悟空的七窍，又按摩揉擦，不一会

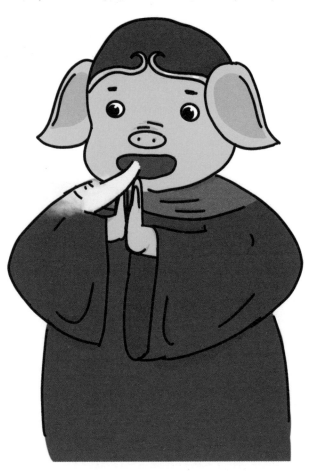

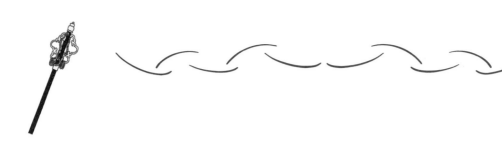
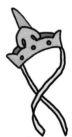

儿，悟空便清醒了。

　　悟空沉思道："龙王的水奈何不了三昧真火，如今恐怕只有观音菩萨能收服他了。我这就去南海求见菩萨！"

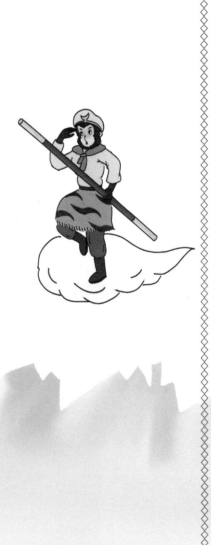

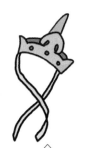
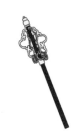

　　观音得知事情的来龙去脉后，将整整一海的水收进手中的玉净瓶里，同悟空速速赶往火云洞。只见那净瓶一倒，三昧真火立刻被大水熄灭，火云洞前也成了汪洋大海。

　　眼见法阵被破，红孩儿只能亲自出战。但那红孩儿除了这三昧真火，其他本领皆敌不过悟空，不一会儿便落败了。观音菩萨念红孩儿聪慧有本领，并且良性未泯，存有孝心，就收红孩儿为善财童子，带到南海修行去了。

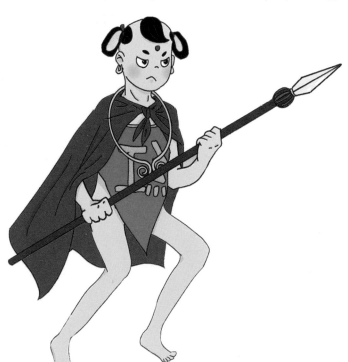

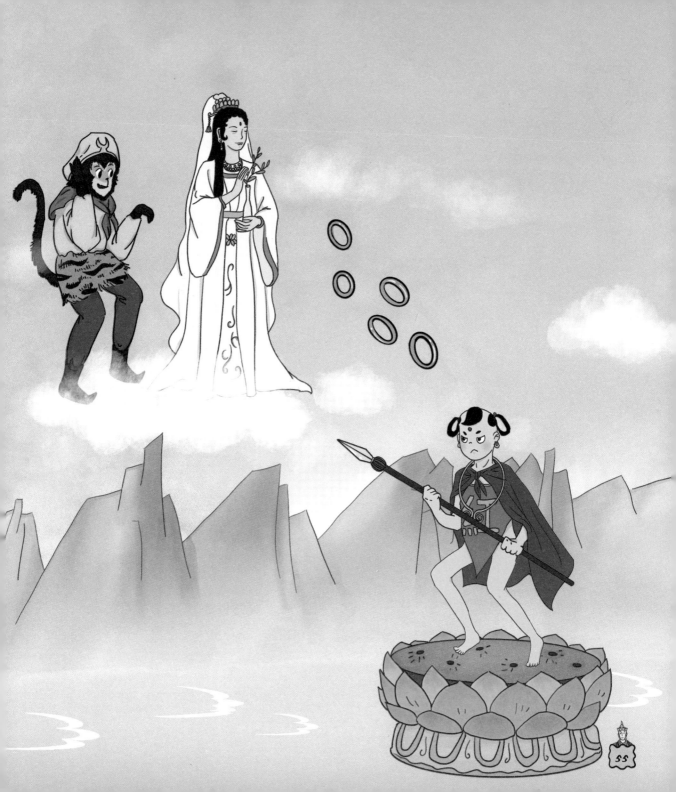

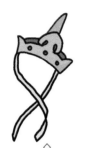
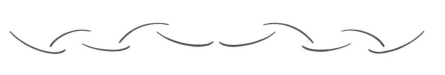
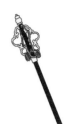
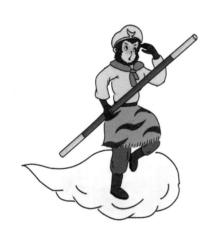
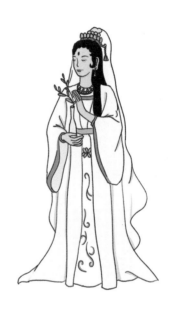
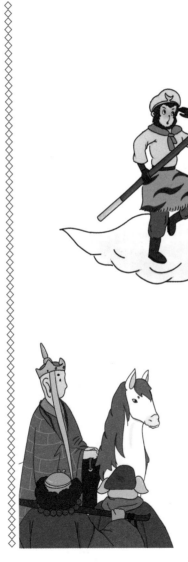

悟空告别了观音，救出师父，一把火烧了火云洞，然后师徒四人继续向西天走去。

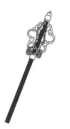
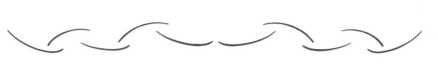
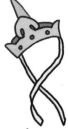

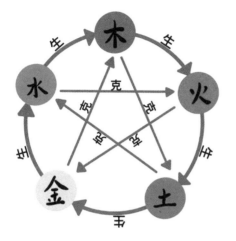

五行相生相克学说

　　"五行相生"指两类属性不同的事物之间存在有序的促进、助长关系。具体为木生火，火生土，土生金，金生水，水生木。

　　"五行相克"与"五行相生"相反，指五行之间有序的克制作用。具体为木克土，土克水，水克火，火克金，金克木。

神医孙悟空

西行路漫漫。这日，唐僧师徒四人来到朱紫国。听说这里的国王身患重病，太医用尽了办法，国王却久治不愈，只好悬赏求医。孙悟空一向爱凑热闹，仗着自己本领高强，二话不说，过去便揭了皇榜。太医们好像见了大救星一样，忙请他们进宫为国王诊治。

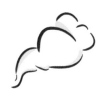

　　国王躺在床上，看起来神情疲倦，郁郁寡欢。他无精打采地问悟空："不知道神医准备如何给寡人诊治？"

　　悟空摸着下巴，摇头晃脑地说："当然是望闻问切了。"

　　国王好奇地问："什么是望闻问切呢？"

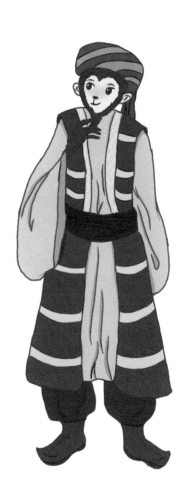

　　悟空回答："望，就是让俺老孙瞧瞧您的气色，观察陛下您的舌象。闻呢，就是听听陛下的声息，闻一闻陛下身上的气味。问，自然是询问陛下的病情。切嘛，陛下您贵为天子，我不能直接为您摸脉，只好悬丝诊脉了。"

　　国王又问："这悬丝诊脉又是何物？"

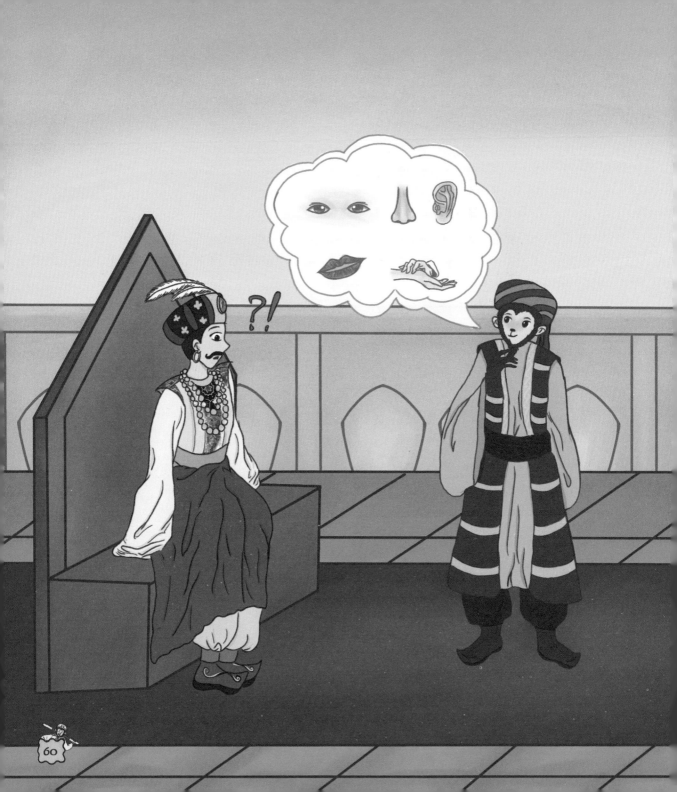

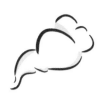

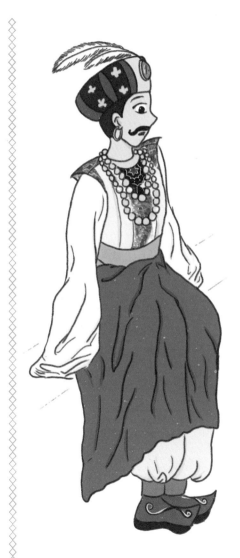

　　悟空拔下三根毫毛，变作三根丝线，让太监把丝线依次绑在国王左手腕上的寸、关、尺部位，说："这便是悬丝诊脉。"

　　悟空隔着帘子，拿着线头，先用自己右手大拇指托着三根线中的一根，食指摸寸脉，再用中指摸关脉，无名指摸尺脉。随后，他又让太监如法炮制，把丝线系在国王的右手腕上，自己改用左手把脉。

　　悟空沉思了片刻，胸有成竹地说："从陛下脉象可以看出，您脾胃虚寒，心中郁结，体内有饮食积滞。这病是因长时间的担惊受怕和思念过度而起，我说得对不对？"国王听了连连点头。

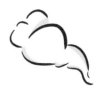

悟空捋捋胡子，笑嘻嘻地说：
"您的病叫作'双鸟失群'之证。
放心吧，这种小病对我来说简直
是小菜一碟！"

众官啧啧称奇，七嘴八舌地
问道："神僧长老，这'双鸟失
群'之证，我们闻所未闻，究竟
是个什么病呀？"

悟空笑道："曾经有雌雄二
鸟，原先在一处同飞，每日形影
不离，忽然被暴风骤雨惊散，雌
雄不得相见，昼思夜想，这不是
双鸟失群吗？"

众人听了，纷纷称赞悟空是
神医再世。

国王大喜，连忙从床上坐起
身子，请悟空帮他开药方治病。

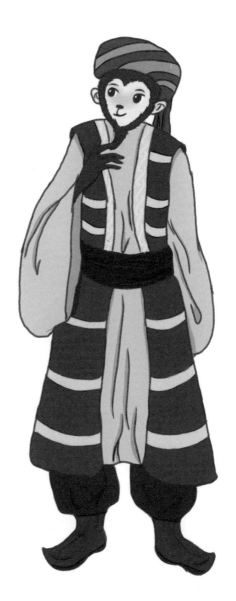

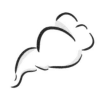

悟空想了想，说："要想治好病，您需要给我准备好八百零八种药材，每种各三斤，和制药的工具一起送到驿馆我的住处！"

一旁的御医吃了一惊，十分不解："自古以来，从没听说过哪个方子会用到这么多的药啊！"

悟空一甩手，装出一副不高兴的样子，斥责道："怎么，你们嫌多吗？没有一成不变的药方，只要合适就能治病。你们要是不肯找，大不了俺老孙罢手不管了！"这可把国王急坏了，一叠声地吩咐道："不多，不多！便是要八千零八种、八万零八种，寡人也给！快，快去给神医准备！"

没过多久，驿馆门前就来了好几辆大车，每辆车里都装了满满的药材，隔着几条街都能闻

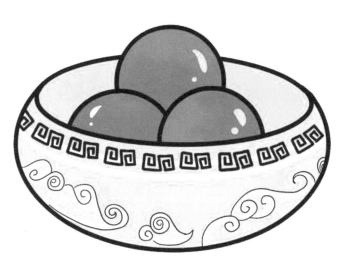

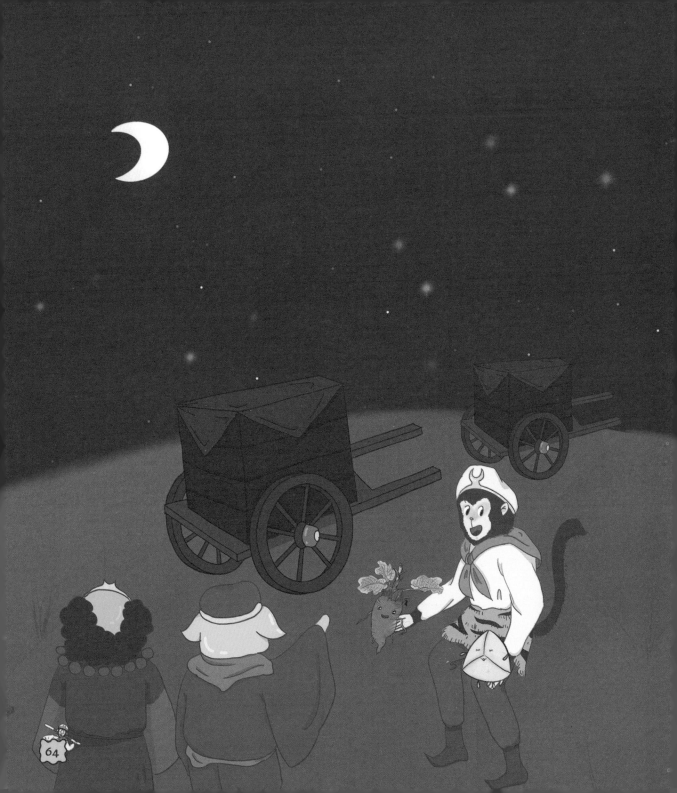

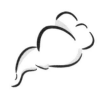

见草药的香味。

晚上，悟空叫来八戒和沙僧一起帮忙制药，却只在八百零八味药材中取出两样：大黄、巴豆各一两。

沙僧问："大黄大苦大寒，陛下病了这么久，身体肯定已经很虚弱，怎么能用泻下力量这么强的药呢？"

悟空答道："三弟你不懂，这大黄能够利痰顺气、泻下攻积，正好把陛下腹内的污秽清一清！"

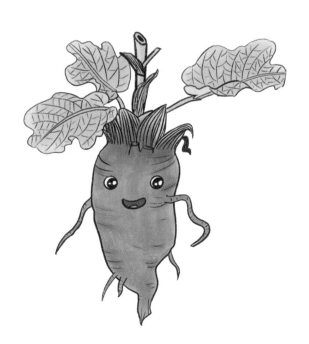

八戒指着巴豆说："这药我认得，是峻猛的泻药，可不能乱用啊！"

悟空狡黠一笑："八戒啊，说你是呆子，你还真是个呆子！此药破结宣肠，能理心膨水胀，既能

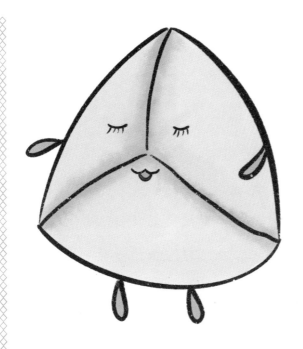

祛寒，又能通便，哪是乱用？正是因为太医们畏手畏脚，不敢大胆用药，我才讨要来这么多药材，免得他们猜出我的用意又来阻拦，多麻烦呀！"

八戒、沙僧恍然大悟，师兄弟三人忙得热火朝天。沙僧将大黄研磨成细粉，八戒将巴豆去壳去膜，捶去油妻，碾为细末，悟空又要他们去取半盏锅底的灰和半盏马尿回来。这下沙僧和八戒又不懂了，怎么能让人吃锅灰，喝马尿呢？

悟空解释道："锅灰名为百草霜，能调百病。至于这马尿嘛，可不是普通的马尿，咱们的白龙马可是龙变化的，尿里面有仙气呢！"

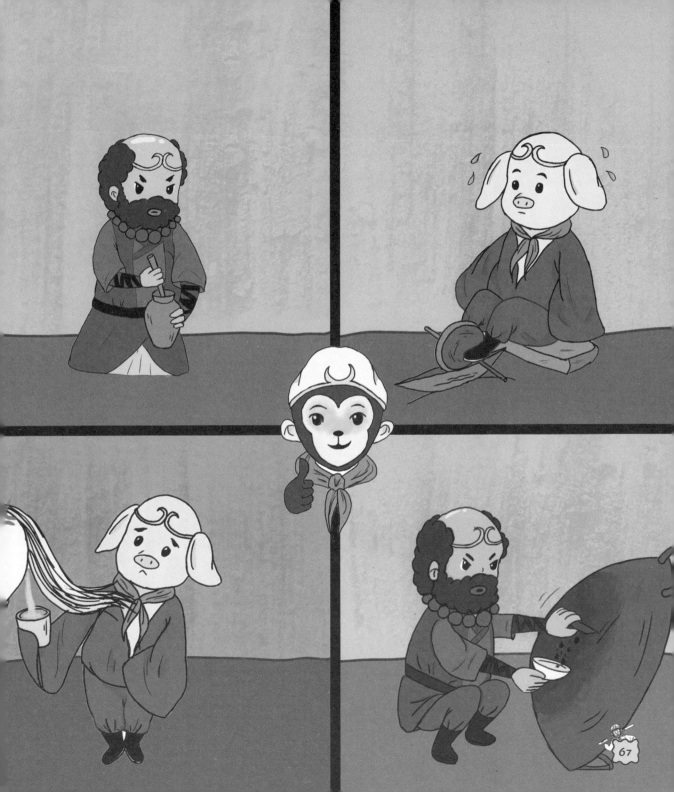

悟空把马尿和药粉混合，做成三颗大药丸，称之为"乌金丹"。

　　第二天，三粒药丸被送到宫里，又按悟空的要求，让太监接了干净的雨水作为药引。国王和着雨水吃下药丸，不一会儿就有了便意，把污秽、病根排了个一干二净，顿时精神抖擞，什么病也没有了。

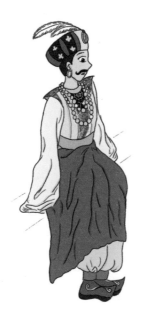

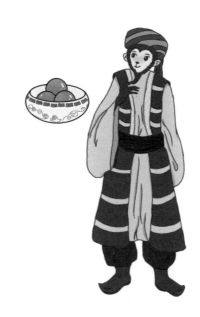

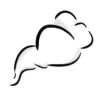

后　续

　　国王感激悟空的救命之恩，举办盛大的宴会招待师徒四人。吃饭时，悟空问国王："俺老孙只知道陛下您得的是相思病，却不知道陛下究竟有什么心事？"一问才知，原来三年前，国王的妻子被妖怪掳走，自此忧心忡忡，患了怪病。常言道："解铃还须系铃人，心病还需心药医。"孙悟空急人所难，把王后救了回来，让一对佳偶破镜重圆，国王的病才算是真真正正地治好了，师徒四人也安心告辞西行。

望闻问切

"四诊"指的是望、闻、问、切，古称"诊法"，是中医诊断疾病的四种方法。传统中医认为，无论什么疾病，都有特定的表象，通过四诊法的诊断，可以帮助医生根据表象辨明疾病，从而更好地治疗患者。

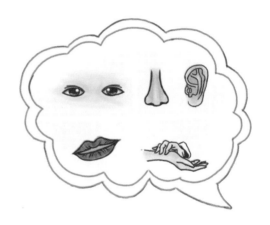

"望诊"是指观察患者的神色形态、舌象、头面、五官、大小便等。"闻诊"是指听患者的说话、咳嗽、喘息等声音，并且嗅患者发出的异常气味（比如口臭、体臭等）或者排出物的气味。"问诊"是指医生询问患者自己所感受到的不适症状以及病史等。"切诊"是指医生用手诊脉，或按压腹部等部位看是否有硬块或者其他症状。"四诊合参"指结合所有的诊断手法，全面地判断病情，这是中医诊断的重要原则。

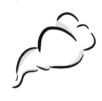

脉诊

　　中医的脉诊又叫把脉，是通过长期医疗实践经验总结出来的诊断方法。医生用手指按压患者的脉搏来了解病情，比如感受脉搏的浅深、粗细、快慢、强弱、流畅度、节律等。脉象与疾病的病位、性质等密切相关。

　　最常见的脉诊部位位于腕部桡动脉。正常人的脉象应该是不慢不快，从容和缓，柔和有力，流畅均匀，节律一致，一次平缓呼吸的时间，脉搏跳动4～5次。一般来讲，年龄越小，

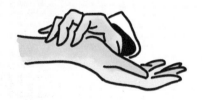

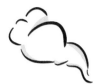

脉搏越快。婴儿每分钟脉搏120次；五六岁的儿童，每分钟脉搏90～110次。把脉的时间一般在1分钟以上，最好是3～5分钟。诊脉时，医生要全神贯注。在把脉过程中大家要尽量保持安静哦，不要乱动，否则会影响把脉的结果。

脉诊虽然感觉高深莫测，其实通过正确的指导和反复的训练，是可以被掌握的。

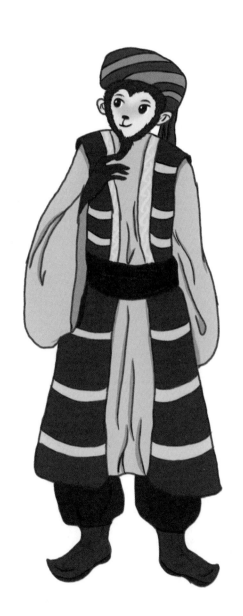

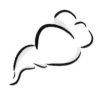

大　黄

　　大黄其实是多种蓼（liǎo）科大黄属的多年生植物的合称。将植物的根茎风干、烘干或切片晒干，就成了中药材大黄。大黄具有泻下攻积、清热泻火、解毒止血、活血化瘀的功效，有"药中张飞"之称，甚至被人认为是"虎狼之药"，由此可见大黄的功效十分峻猛。

　　孙悟空用大黄给国王通便，排出体内积累的杂物、毒素。一般而言，医生给身体虚弱的患者开的药都比较温和，而孙悟空大胆地给国王吃大黄，其实具有一定的风险，太医们如果知道是万万不敢给国王用的。

巴　豆

中药用的巴豆是巴豆树的干燥成熟果实，这种植物喜阳光，怕寒冻，生长在温暖湿润的地区。巴豆不仅和大黄一样能让人腹泻，还有大毒！即便是孙悟空，使用巴豆也需要炮制得当、用量准确才行。

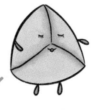

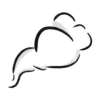

丸　剂

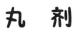

　　丸剂，是将药材磨成细末，用米、水或者米糊、面糊、酒、醋、药汁等揉成丸状。制成药丸可以缓和某些峻猛药品的药性。孙悟空就是用马尿使药末成丸，降低大黄和巴豆的毒性，使药物作用缓和而持久，采取了峻药缓治的方法。

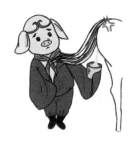
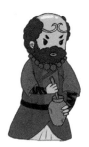
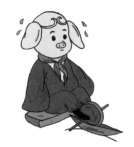

后 记

　　跟随师徒四人的西行历程告一段落，相信我们可爱的小读者也在西游途中收获了不少中医药知识。

　　然而，一本《西游记》中的中医药知识只是中医学宝库的一角，更多的中医药知识需要我们一起去探索和发掘。

　　亲爱的小读者们，中医药是一座伟大的宝库，希望你们能够畅游其中，尽情体会中医药的神奇魅力！

王珊珊

2022 年 11 月

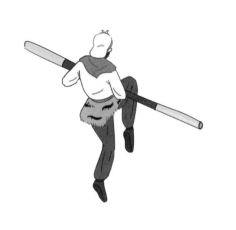
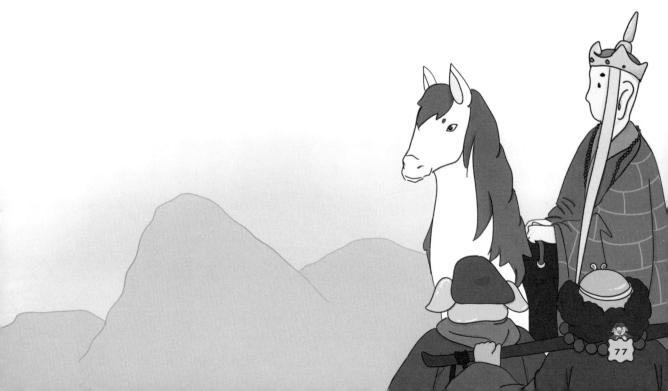

JOURNEY

TO

THE WEST

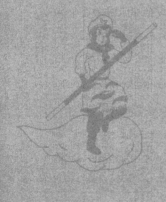

Gathering Herbs from the
Mountain of Flowers and Fruit

Once upon a time, at the edge of the Aolai country, there was a place called the Mountain of Flowers and Fruit. A magic rock had stood alone on top of the mountain. One day, the rock split open, and a stone monkey jumped out. Just like other monkeys, the stone monkey fed from plants, drank from springs, picked flowers and looked for food in the mountain.

At that time, the weather was so hot that monkeys ran to play in the cool water. The stone monkey came along with them. The monkeys were surprised to see the waterfall, the source of stream, and everyone was eager to put in a word. "Whoever can jump through and come back alive will be our king!" they decided. All the monkeys looked at one another, but no one was brave enough to have a try. Suddenly, a voice called out, "I'll do it!" It was the stone monkey who came out. He took a deep breath and leaped into the waterfall. He landed in an iron bridge, opening his eyes. He noticed some big letters: HAPPY LAND OF THE MOUNTAIN OF FLOWERS AND

FRUIT, CAVE HEAVEN OF THE WATER CURTAIN. The stone monkey was beside himself with joy. He rushed away, crouched, and leaped back through the waterfall.

All the other monkeys crowded around him, asking, "What's it like in there? How deep is the water?" "We're in luck! I found a perfect home for all of us. Follow me!" The monkeys grinned. They jumped through after him joyfully. They kept their words, bowing to the stone monkey, and called him the Handsome Monkey King.

Many years went by. During those days, under the leadership of the Handsome Monkey King, the monkeys and apes played in the forest and stream, and every night slept safely in their caves.

In spring they picked flowers for food and drink,
In summer they lived off fruit.
In autumn they gathered nuts,
They got through the winter on Huangjing.

One day, the Handsome Monkey King directed other monkeys to set out to pick peaches and dig out yams, cook Huangjing and some other seeds. The monkeys ate with relish and asked the Handsome Monkey King, "What is it, my king?" "It is Huangjing. It can strengthen the body, and good for the spleen and kidney. If Uncle Monkey feels sore and weak on the waist and knees, it will be helpful." At that moment, a cry was heard in the distance. It was a baby monkey with swollen leg. He couldn't sleep well, kept crying, and refused to eat anything. The Handsome Monkey King fed him with Yimi and Fuling, trying to comfort him, "Calm down, poor little thing. It is nothing but edema, a common disease. These two herbs will do you good." After taking the herbs, the swelling in the little monkey's legs gradually disappeared. He could eat and sleep well, and played with other monkeys happily as before.

◆ Huangjing (Solomon's seed) ◆

Huangjing can reinforce qi to replenish yin, and benefit the spleen, lung and kidney.

According to the TCM theory, the waist is the house of kidney. As age creeps up, seniors may suffer from kidney deficiency, and that's why our grandparents are usually seen with lumbar and leg pain.

In this story, eating Huangjing relieves Uncle Monkey's pain. Drinking water with pieces of Huangjing can replenish blood. But it's improper to take in too much in case it increases the burden of spleen for digestion.

◆ Fuling (Poria cocos) ◆

Fuling can benefit the spleen and heart, and induce urination effectively. The baby monkey ate Fuling, which helped him discharge the extra water in his body by promoting urination, and relieve edema. But we should pay attention to the dosage when it is applied to children.

◆ Yiyiren (Coix seed) ◆

Yiyiren, is the Yiyiren seed in our daily diet. Yiyiren is a traditional Chinese food for health preservation.

Yiyiren and Fuling are highly praised for their function of invigorating the spleen. The spleen is one of the five zang-organs, with transportation and transformation as its main function. People living in wet areas often use Yiyiren and Fuling to make soup or porridge to remove dampness from the body. It is recorded in the ancient medical books that taking Yiyiren regularly for a long time can make our skin white and fair.

Trouble in Heaven

Monkey lived a happy life in Mountain of Flowers and Fruit. He was healthy and strong, and learned many magical skills from his teacher. After that, he made troubles in the Dragon Palace and the Land of Darkness. Then Dragon King and Judge of the Dead came to Jade Emperor and made complains about Monkey. Great White Planet Venus (Tai Bai Jin Xing) said to Jade Emperor why not give Monkey a job in Heaven, then they could keep a close eye on Monkey, so he would not cause any trouble. Jade Emperor agreed and sent Monkey to feed horses. Monkey soon found that he was in the lowest position in Heaven. He was in a great anger and returned to the Mountain of Flowers and Fruit, and proclaimed himself the Great Sage Equal to Heaven (Qi Tian Da Sheng).

Jade Emperor heard that Monkey came back to the Mountain of Flowers and Fruit. In his fury he asked King Li, a Heaven King with a Pagoda in Hand, and his third son Ne Zha, to lead the soldiers to arrest Monkey. But they all failed. Great White Planet Venus had an idea. He said, "If that monkey likes this name, then give him this name.

It's just a name without any real power". Jade Emperor thought it was not a bad idea and sent Great White Planet Venus to make peace with Monkey.

Monkey agreed with that pleasantly and returned to Heaven with him. After a long time, Jade Emperor worried that Monkey had nothing to do and he would make some troubles. So he put Monkey in charge of the Royal Peach Garden. But since Monkey was not a well-behaved one, he ate all the bigger peaches during the Peach Festival held by Queen Mother. He made a havoc during the festival and finally made himself in a big trouble. He then came back to the Mountain of Flowers and Fruit again. After hearing all of this, Jade Emperor erupted into fury and sent soldiers to take this horrible monkey back to Heaven.

Monkey was tied on the Monsters Killing Platform, but couldn't be harmed a little neither by swords nor by water and fire. Gods and spirits could not get him hurt at all. At that time, Lord Lao Zi (Tai Shang Lao Jun) had a plan, and said, "Your Majesty, that monkey was a birth of Heaven and Earth, and ate a lot of royal peaches and elixir. His body has already been hard as a diamond and cannot be destroyed. Why not put him into my furnace which I use to make elixir to ruin him." The angry Jade Emperor immediately agreed to the suggestion.

Monkey was put into the furnace, and driven to rush here and there by the high temperature. The boys who made the fire on tried their best to keep it burning, hoping the horrible monkey would be destroyed as soon as possible.

The fire kept burning for forty-nine days, and finally there was no noise in the furnace. The Lord Lao Zi opened the lid of it with great confidence, but saw something just jumped out. Oh, it's Monkey. But Monkey should have been burned up and destroyed!

Actually, it is the Eight Trigrams Furnace, which is made up of the Eight Trigrams-Qian, Kan, Gen, Zhen, Sun, Li, Kun, and Dui. As a saying goes, one door closes, another door opens. Monkey jumped up and down in the furnace, and finally jumped into a place named "Palace of Sun". Because Sun was the wind, and there was no fire but a lot of smoke in that position. Monkey stayed there for forty-nine days, and he consequently got fire eyes with golden pupils.

Monkey leaped out and kicked it down. He took his

Golden cudgel out and beat soldiers and gods to get to the Cloud Palace.

Jade Emperor had no idea, and could only send someone to the Western Paradise to ask Buddha to come here for help. But Monkey turned a blind eye to him.

Buddha was calm. He smiled and spread his hand wide, saying, "Let's make a deal. If you jump off my hand, I will make you take the place of Jade Emperor to rule Heaven."

Monkey could travel about hundreds of thousands of miles by one leap, so he was very confident. He said, "A word spoken is past recalling! I'm leaving and you cannot break your promise." Then he leaped and traveled fast.

After a long time, he saw five enormous pillars, and then stopped. He thought, "these pillars must be the support of the sky, and this place must be the end of the world."

Monkey thought that no one could prove he once came here, so he pulled out one hair and turned it into a large brush. He wrote on the middle pillar "Great Sage Equal to Heaven was here". Then he peed at the foot of the first pillar, and went back to Buddha. Monkey yelled, "Buddha, you must keep your promise. Now, ask Jade

Emperor come here and give his position to me."

But Buddha said he actually never left his hand. Monkey wasn't convinced and asked Buddha to see the thing he left at the end of the world. Then Buddha asked Monkey to see his middle finger and smelled the flavor of his thumb. Monkey opened his eyes wide and only saw the words he had written on the middle finger, and also smelled the odor of his pee.

Monkey said in surprise, "No, you must be kidding! You are playing a trick on me. I wrote these words on the pillar supporting the sky, but why are these words on your finger? Let me go to check it."

Monkey wanted to run away, but Buddha turned his hand over and pushed Monkey out of the Gate of Western Paradise. He turned his fingers into a giant mountain chain named the Five Elements Mountain. Five Elements refer to Metal, Wood, Water, Fire and Earth. Monkey was held under that mountain and could not move.

When Buddha returned to the Western Paradise, he passed by the Five Elements Mountain. He said to the gods who would keep an eye on Monkey, "Five hundred years later, someone will come here and save him."

◆ Five Elements（Wu Xing）◆

The mountain that traps Monkey named the Five Elements Mountain. It's changed from the fingers of Buddha. It's a mountain chain representing five elements, i.e. metal, wood, water, fire and earth.

Five elements is a term in Traditional Chinese Medicine. It's a concept of ancient Chinese philosophy in exploring nature. It divides everything in nature into five elements. These elements have their own functions and attributes.Wood is characterized by growing and developing freely; fire, warming and rising; earth, bearing and breeding; metal, descending and restraining; and water, moistening and cooling.

When applied to the human body, five elements represent the five zang-organs. Metal, wood, water, fire and earth correspond to the lung, liver, kidney, heart and spleen respectively.

Good Medicine for Wind Eye

Monk saved Monkey from the Five Elements Mountain, and accepted Pig as another disciple. They worked hard day and night in their journey to the west.

When they were crossing a mountain, a tiger leapt out. He yelled, "I'm Tiger Commander, serving Great Yellow Wind King. The king asked me to patrol the mountain. Who are you, monks?" Monk and his disciples explained and asked him to let them go.

But the monster had heard of the rumor that eating Monk's flesh could be living forever. "If I could capture the monk, I would not only gain a reward from the King, but also get a bite of his flesh," he thought. So he fought with them without explanation, but could not beat them down.

He then peeled off his skin, and turned into a storm. When he ran away, he noticed Monk waiting there alone, and grabbed him as a gift for Great Yellow Wind King.

However, Monkey and Pig couldn't see through the monster's trick. They hit the fake tiger together, but the fake tiger changed into a puff of black smoke. At that moment, they realized the monster had tricked them. They came back to search for Monk but only to find it was too late.

Monkey and Pig chased the monster into the mountain, until they found a gate. When Pig was looking after the horse and luggage, Monkey went to fight with the monsters inside. The leader of them, Great Yellow Wind King fought with Monkey over thirty rounds but had no clear winner, so he blew to Monkey immediately— that was his trick. Monkey was suddenly hit by stabbing pain in his eyes, and he couldn't see anything. He had no choice but to flee from the battle, and the monster also went back to his cave.

Monkey and Pig found a house under the slope. They knocked at the door, and an old man walked out, giving them a warm welcome. In fact, the old man was a Buddha, waiting here to help them, but Monkey and Pig didn't know it. Monkey kept rubbing his eyes, so the old man asked, "What's wrong with you?"

"Do you know what disease it is, grandpa? I was blown on by a monster, and my eyes have been aching and tears flowing." Monkey said angrily.

"It is wind eye," the old man explained, "The monster

blew a breath of wind and heat on you. You must cure it completely, or it will get worse later."

Monkey was so worried that he scratched his head and asked, "I can't live without my eyes! What can I do?"

The old man brought out a tiny bottle, and said, "It is 'Three Flowers Nine Seeds Ointment'. There are some vision-improving herbs in it, such as chrysanthemum flowers, cassia seeds and wolfberry fruits. It can cure all discomfort of the eyes." Then, he put a tiny amount in Monkey's eyes, and told him to keep the eyes closed until tomorrow morning. He could go to sleep without any worry, because everything would be back to normal then.

When Monkey opened his eyes the next morning, he happily said, "It certainly is good ointment— I can see far, far more clearly than ever!"

◆ Six Excesses ◆

There are six kinds of climatic changes in nature, including wind, cold, summer-heat, dampness, dryness and fire. When they change excessively and become adverse environmental conditions, they are called six excesses, then diseases occur. For example, human body can resist the summer-heat and will not get ill, although the weather of summer is hot. But if you expose yourself to the sun for a long time, the heat will turn to be heat evil, which can cause heatstroke, dizziness, nausea, and even coma. The characteristics of six excesses are different, which is helpful for the doctors to identify the cause of diseases from the symptoms.

Wind evil is the main reason for Monkey's eyes ache. Wind evil is the first one in six excesses, because it can cause many diseases, or hurt our body combined with other evils. In this story, Monkey is injured by wind evil mixed up with fire evil. So we are suggested to have daily exercise to keep away from the attack of wind evil.

Delicious Manfruits

After curing the eyes, Monkey defeated Great Yellow Wind King. They rescued Monk and continued their journey. Then, Monk accepted Sand as his disciple. One day, they arrived at a mountain, and there was a Taoist temple called Wuzhuang Temple. They stopped to spend the night in the temple. Two Taoist boys came out to welcome them. "We are sorry we did not welcome you properly," they said. "Our master said you were his old friend of previous birth. You can stay and feel at home, venerable Master."

The two boys treated Monk with great politeness, and picked manfruits for him. However, the shape of manfruit was like a baby. Monk was afraid of it, so he rejected. The boys just returned to their room and shared the manfruits.

Unexpectedly, Pig saw through the whole thing. He told Monkey of it, and wondered, "Why did the boys call the manfruit as 'the fruit for the gods'? Is it delicious?" "The manfruit is really a good thing, and anyone who can eat it lives to a great old age." Monkey said. Pig greedily pleaded, "What a good fruit! Brother, you are the best among us. Why don't you pick some and share with us?"

Monkey took the golden rod that the boys had used and went to the garden to pick manfruits. He jumped upon the tree branch, tapping the manfruit, but the fruit disappeared as soon as they tumbled down onto the ground. Monkey believed it was the garden deity— the god of the earth— who had stolen his manfruits, so he forced him to come out.

"You get me wrong, Great Sage," the deity said, "These fruits have something to do with the knowledge of Five Elements. They only fear the Five Elements. If they meet metal, they fall; if they meet fire, they are burnt; and if they meet earth, they go into it. If you tap them you have to use a golden rod, otherwise they won't drop; and when you knock them down, you must catch them in a bowl padded with silk." Monkey did as he said, knocking down three manfruits.

He took the fruit back, and shared them with his brothers. Sand said, "This sweet fruit really quenches my thirst. Thank you, brother!" But after a short while, the two boys found manfruits had been stolen. They abused and cursed Monk and his disciples. Annoyed by this, Monkey smashed the manfruit trees. Zhen Yuan Zi, the owner of the Taoist temple, who happened to come back, was furious about it. But he remembered the friendship with Monk, so he ordered Monkey to bring the tree back to life, and only in this way could he forgive them.

Monkey asked everywhere, but no one know how to revive the manfruit trees. Finally, he had to go to Bodhisattva for help. Fortunately, the water in Bodhisattva's jade bottle could save every plant.

Monkey came back to the temple together with Bodhisattva. Bodhisattva asked Monkey and his brothers to straighten the trees and bury the roots with soil. After that, Bodhisattva recited a spell, watering the manfruit trees with the water in her jade bottle. Sooner, the leaves of the trees turned green again, and the fruits grew out, as lush as before.

Zhen Yuan Zi also turned his anger into joy. He immediately asked the boys to knock down ten manfruits and entertained his guests. At this time, Monk realized that the manfruit was indeed a fruit, so he also ate one. After the banquet, Zhen Yuan Zi sent them on to their journey.

◆ Manfruit (Ginseng Fruit) ◆

Unlike the baby-like manfruit in the novel, which can prolong human's life, the ginseng fruit in reality is round. It is a kind of vegetable or fruit with all-sided nutritional health value. It tastes crisp, sweet and juicy with a delicate smell. Its functions include lowering blood sugar and blood lipid, improving memory and sleep, etc.

The Fight with Red Boy

When Monk and his disciples arrived at a rocky mountain, a sudden wind from the mountain made them unable to open their eyes. After the wind stopped, Monk had disappeared. Monkey looked around, and found a stone tablet on which big letters were carved, FIRE-WIND CAVE. Inside was a monster called Red Boy, who believed that eating Monk could make him live forever, so he captured Monk with evil wind.

Monkey, Pig and Sand went to the cave immediately, and challenged Red Boy inside. The little devils set the carts out in the order of the Five Elements— metal, wood, water, fire and earth. The flames are burning like red clouds.

Monkey's magical powers were really great. Making a spell with his fingers, he rushed into the flames to chase the demon. However, the cave was full of smoke. Reluctantly, Monkey came back and asked for his brothers' opinion.

"The only reason you can't beat him is his fire. If you take my advice, you may catch him easily by using the principle of relationship between the elements," said

Sand. "According to this principle, we'll have to beat fire with water." Monkey said cheerfully, "You're right. I'll go and borrow some dragon soldiers from the oceans to bring water to douse the devil fire."

The four dragon kings came with Monkey, and brought a splendid rainstorm. Heavy though it was, the downpour could not stop Red Boy's fire. The water could only put out ordinary fires, but not this evil fire.

Monkey was worried about the safety of Monk, so he rushed into the fire again. Seeing Monkey, Red Boy blew a cloud of smoke straight into his face. The flames and smoke had made Monkey unbearably hot, so he plunged straight into the stream to put out the flames, not realizing that the shock of the cold water would make the fire attack his heart, and even drove his three souls out of him.

Pig and Sand saved Monkey from the river, but Monkey was curled up, unable to stretch his limbs and as cold as ice all over. Pig warmed Monkey up by rubbing vigorously with the palms of his hands, covered his seven orifices, and gave him a massage. The shock of the cold water had blocked the qi in Monkey's abdomen, leaving him unable to speak. Thanks to Pig's massage and rubbing,

Monkey woke up. He decided to turn to Bodhisattva for help.

Bodhisattva came with Monkey, using the water in her jade bottle to put out the evil fire. Red Boy could only go out to fight in person, but he was not Monkey's equal. He was defeated soon. Bodhisattva thought he was an intelligent boy of capability, and his nature was not bad, so she took Red Boy as disciple and allowed him to go with her.

Monkey parted with Bodhisattva and rescued Monk. He set fire to the demon cave. Then Monk together with his disciples continued their journey to the West.

◆ The Theory of the Inter-generation and Inter-restriction between Five Elements ◆

The inter-generation means that one of the five elements promotes, supports and generates another element. Wood generates fire, fire generates earth, earth generates metal, metal generates water, and water generates wood.

The inter-restriction is opposite with the inter-generation. It means one of the five elements restricts and controls another element. Wood restricts earth, earth restricts water, water restricts fire, fire restricts metal, and metal restricts wood.

Doctor Monkey

One day, Monk and his disciples came to the Land of Purpuria. They heard the king of it was seriously ill. Although every method had been tried on him by the royal doctors, it seems he didn't get well. He issued a notice looking for highly skilled doctors. Monkey took down the royal notice, and soon he was invited to the palace to see the king, because the royal doctors thought he was their savior.

Lying on bed, the king looked tired and depressed. "What's your plan, doctor?" said the king downheartedly.

"By observing, listening and smelling, inquiry and touching." Monkey touched his chin and answered.

"What does it mean?" The king asked.

"Observing is to have a look at your complexion and tongue. Listening is to listen to your voice and breath. Smelling is to smell your body odor. Inquiry is to ask about your illness. Touching is to feel your pulses. But considering your status, your Majesty, I will take your pulses by threads."

"How to feel the pulses by threads?" asked the king.

Monkey pulled out three hairs and turned them into three golden threads. He asked the servants to tie these threads to the king's left wrist at the cun, guan and chi sections respectively.

Monkey sat behind the screen. He took these threads and held one thread by his thumb pulp of his right hand. He used his forefinger to felt the pulse at the cun section, his middle finger to feel the pulse at the guan section, and his fourth finger to feel the chi pulse. And then Monkey felt the pulse of the king's right hand with his left hand.

A moment later, he said confidently, "There is food retention in your body, and deficiency-cold in your spleen and stomach. You feel depressed as well. Your majesty's disease is due to a long time of fear and excessive thinking, am I right?"

The king nodded.

"The condition is the one known as 'a pair of birds parted'. It's not a big deal, just take it easy." Monkey smiled.

All the officials were surprised and came forward to ask, "What does that mean, holy monk?"

"It's when a cock and a hen who were flying together

are suddenly separated by a violent storm," said Monkey with a smile again. "They can't see each other. The hen misses the cock and the cock misses the hen. Isn't that 'a pair of birds parted'?"

"He is a real holy monk!" The officials all cried out.

The king was overjoyed and got up from bed to ask Monkey to give him a prescription.

"Your majesty, if you want to cure your disease, you need to prepare three pounds of each 808 Chinese herbs together with the medicine processing tools, and send them to the hostel." Monkey said after a while.

Other doctors were so surprised and asked, "I haven't heard that one could use so much medicine in one prescription. Are you serious?"

Monkey shook off his hands, pretending to be unhappy and scolded, "Oh? Are these too much? There is no fixed prescription. If you don't do as I said, I'll leave your king alone!"

The king was so nervous, saying, "That's no problem! Even if the holy monk wanted 8008 herbs or more, I'd like to give them to him! Quickly, get them ready for the holy monk!"

Soon after, here came several carriages full of herbs and finally stopped in front of the hostel. The flavor of herbs could be smelled by people in a long distance.

In the evening, Monkey asked Pig and Sand to help him process drugs. He only picked up one ounce of rhubarb (Da Huang) and one ounce of croton (Ba Dou).

"Rhubarb has a bitter taste and a cold nature and isn't poisonous," said Sand. "But perhaps it's bad for the king since he is now so weak after a long illness."

"That's what you don't know, brother," Monkey said. "This drug moves phlegm, and helps clear the evil out of the body."

Pig pointed at the croton seeds and said, "I know it. It's a powerful laxative. You must be very careful about how you use it."

"Brother," Monkey replied, "This drug can smooth bowels, remove water retention and help doing a poo. And that's just what the king needs."

"Those doctors were too frightened to use medicine, so I asked these herbs from them. I wanted to avoid them asking too much and coming to stop us." said Monkey.

Hearing that, Sand and Pig set their heart into stomach

and got busy. Sand ground the rhubarb to a fine powder with a roller, while Pig shelled and peeled the croton seeds, then took the poisonous oil out of them, and finally grounded them to a fine powder. After that, Monkey said, "Take this and add some soot from a cooking pot, Pig. And Sand, fetch me half a bowl of our horse's piss." Then his brothers were confused, How can you give a human horse's piss to drink and soot to eat?

"The soot from a cooking pot is called 'frost on the flowers'. It helps to treat all kinds of illnesses." said Monkey, "The horse of ours is not an ordinary one. He used to be a dragon in the Western Ocean. His piss can cure any illness you could have."

Finally, Monkey mixed the piss with the powder into a pill called "Black Gold Elixir".

The next day, the three pills were sent to the palace for the king. According to Monkey's request, servants gathered clean rainwater as medicine usher. The king took the pills with the rainwater. After a short time, he went to the toilet several times and released all the filth and sickness.

The king held a feast to thank Monkey. In the feast,

Monkey asked, "I knew you had a lovesickness, but why? What happened?" It turned out that three years ago, the king's wife was kidnapped by a monster, and he had been very worried ever since. As an old saying goes, "it is better for the doer to undo what he has done." Monkey saved the queen, and the king's illness was completely cured. Monk, Monkey, Pig and Sand set out again on their journey.

◆ The Four Examinations ◆

The four examinations or four diagnostic methods refer to observing, listening and smelling, inquiry, and touching. According to TCM theories, no matter what disease it is, it will present with specific manifestations. "Observing" is to have a look at the patient's vitality, complexion, tongue, five sense organs, urine and stool. "Listening and smelling" refers to listen to the patient's speech, cough, wheezing and other sounds, and smell the patient's smelling such as bad breath. "Inquiry" means a doctor asks about the medical history and present feelings of the patient. "Touching" refers to taking the pulses with fingers. The four interconnected steps constitute the whole process of diagnosis of diseases in TCM.

◆ Pulse Diagnosis ◆

Pulse diagnosis or pulse-taking, as a unique diagnostic method since ancient China, is summarized through thousands of years of medical practice. It is a way to know the illness by feeling the depth, width, rate, intensity, uency and tempo of the pulse. It is believed that the pulse condition is significantly related to the location and nature of disease.

Mostly you'll see the pulse is taken at the radial artery of the wrist. The pulse of a healthy person should be calm and gentle, soft yet powerful, smooth and rhythmic. With one smooth breath, the pulse beats four to five times. Generally speaking, kids have faster pulse than adults. An infant has 120 beats every minute. For children aged five to six, the pulse rate is 90 to 110 times. The time of pulse-taking is often more than 1 minute, preferably 3-5 minutes.

During the process, the doctor should pay close attention to the pulse, and the patient had better keep quiet and not move, or the result is not accurate.

Pulse diagnosis seems to be mysterious, but it can actually be mastered after repeated practice under proper guidance.

◆ Dahuang (Rhubarb) ◆

Dahuang is a tall herb. It's often used as a powerful laxative, which can help pass stools. That's why Monkey applied it to the king. The effect of Dahuang is so strong that can drain downward in order to expel toxins from the body.

It is highly bitter in flavor and cold in nature. Generally, the medicine prescribed by doctors to weak patients should be mild medicine. So it was risky for Monkey to apply the rhubarb and croton seeds to the king. Surely the royal doctors would have stopped Monkey if they knew it.

◆ Badou (Croton seed) ◆

Different from Dahuang, Badou is acrid in avor and hot in nature. It can be a dangerous herb, because it can be strong poison and make people have loose bowels if used inappropriately. Even Monkey must process it carefully, and use it with proper dosage.

◆ Pill ◆

Grind the medicinal herbs into fine powder, and knead it into a pill with rice, water or rice paste, batter, liqueur, vinegar or potion. Medicinal herbs made into the form of pills can soften the effects of some powerful ingredients in it, such as the Dahuang and Badou pills made with horse's piss in this story.

译者注：该译文参照了外文出版社 2015 年出版的詹纳尔（W.J.F Jenner）《西游记》英译本 *Journey to the West*。